WHAT IN THE WORLD IS
E-MENTAL HEALTH?

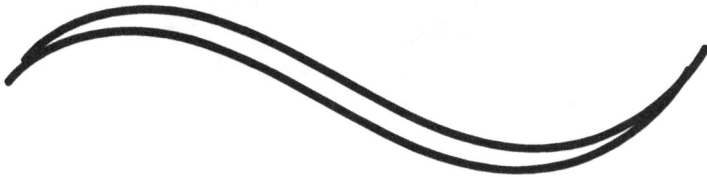

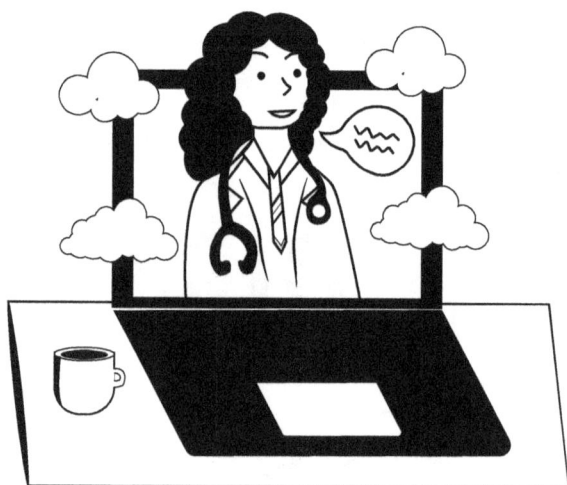

Written and edited by

Austin Mardon, Mohammed Ismael, Massa Mohamed Ali,
Paige Breedon, Hafsa Binte Younus, Jannat Irfan, Abeer
Ansari, Angelina Lam, Maria Ashraf, Madiha Ansari,
Adrienne Lam, Jennifer Pham, Aaliyah Mulla

WHAT IN THE WORLD IS
E-MENTAL HEALTH?

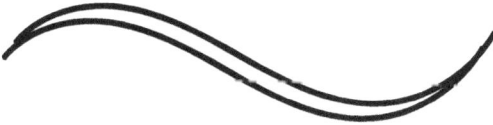

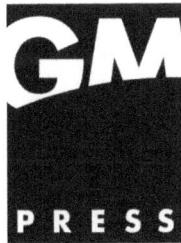

GOLDEN METEORITE PRESS

Typeset and Cover Design by Brianna Purai

ISBN 978-1-77369-235-7
Golden Meteorite Press
103 11919 82 St NW
Edmonton, AB T5B 2W3
www.goldenmeteoritepress.com

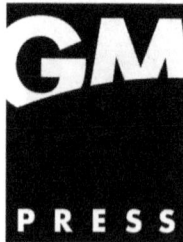

Table of Contents

Background of E-mental Health

Massa Mohamed Ali

Digital transformation and innovation is becoming an increasingly important aspect of today's society. As of April 2021, there are over 4.7 billion active internet users globally, which makes up more than 60% of the world's population. This number is growing daily, with more than 900,000 new users every day ("Global Digital Insights," n.d.). In Canada, the majority of internet users now spend an average of 6 hours on-line per day using multiple devices (Watson, 2021). These technologies are continuously changing the way one engages in daily activities such as shopping, banking, communicating, and seeking health-related information, services, and support. Over the past year, COVID-19 has increased global internet use by 50-70% (Marowits, 2020).

While the internet is commonly used for entertainment, education, and communication purposes, one of its most important uses is in healthcare. Studies among the Canadian population show that the majority of the elderly, youth, mental health service users, and First Nations communities use on-line resources for health support and information (Lal, 2019).

More specifically, on-line mental health support has become increasingly popular and convenient, especially with the effects of the recent pandemic.

According to the Centre for Addiction and Mental Health (CAMH), one in five Canadians experiences a mental illness or addiction problem, with youth aged 15-24 more likely to do so than any other group ("Mental Illness and Addiction: Facts and Statistics," n.d.). Statistics Canada data also shows that since the emergence of COVID-19, fewer Canadians report having excellent or very good mental health – 55% (July 2020) down from 68% (2019). Additionally, COVID-19 further impacted those who were already experiencing poor mental health before the pandemic. Those reporting poor mental health became up to 4 times more likely to report increased substance use. Canadians reported overall increases in their alcohol (16.2%), cannabis (6.1%) and tobacco (4.8%) consumption ("Impacts on Mental Health," 2021).

A digitalized solution to this decrease in mental well-being is the implementation of e-mental health resources. E-mental health involves leveraging the Internet and related technologies such as smartphone apps, websites, and social media to deliver mental health services (Johnson, 2015). While further advancements are still needed for the improvement of Canada's emerging e-mental health resources, over the past decade, this field has made many developments both in Canada and internationally. This book aims to introduce the e-mental health field and its discovery, impacts, significance, benefits, potential, contradictions, and confidentiality.

The concept of e-mental health is derived from the broader term of e-health, which is also referred to as digital health. The World Health Organization (WHO) define e-health as "the cost-effective and secure use of information and communication technologies in support of the health and health-related fields including healthcare, health surveillance and health education, knowledge and research" (Ryu, 2012). This includes Electronic Health Records (EHR), Electronic Medical Records (EMR), health IT systems, virtual healthcare and consultation, telehealth and telemedicine, gerontechnology, m-health, and the use of big data systems. Telemedicine and telehealth connect patients and providers around the world in real time by using video conferencing technologies. This connection allows increased access to health care services and overcomes geographical barriers. Gerontechnology refers to the use of technologies to address the well-being of older adults (Lal, 2019). M-health refers to the use of mobile devices such as smartphones for healthcare, and big data systems use data science techniques to collect and analyse many datasets to ensure a positive impact on patient care outcomes and optimize business processes ("Big Data," n.d.). Essentially, e-mental health is a form of digital health that aims to prevent and treat mental illnesses.

The Mental Health Commission of Canada's (MHCC's) strategy document Changing Directions, Changing

Lives: The Mental Health Strategy for Canada notes that e-mental health can be a solution to the rise in mental health issues (Hatcher, 2014). The document aims to improve mental health outcomes for all Canadians and highlights that "the emerging world of e-health offers new opportunities for interaction and engagement between people who need services and providers. Electronic health records, telemedicine, Internet-based screening and treatment, videoconferencing, and on-line training are all tools that can enhance collaboration, access and skills" (Mental Health Commission of Canada, 2012). E-Mental health can address the gap between the need for better mental health services and the limited capacity to provide conventional treatment services. Digital treatments can be accessible anywhere at any time, eliminate distance barriers, do not include long waiting lists or times, and may not have the same stigma associated with attending an institution.

E-mental health resources can be used in a variety of different ways across the continuum of care and usually target mild to moderate illness severity. They can be used for prevention and early intervention to teach psychological concepts and build resilience. They can also be used as a method of primary treatment to address mild to moderate mental illnesses. E-mental health can also be complementary to another treatment for patients with more severe or chronic mental illnesses (adjunctive treatment). These treatments can later become effective maintenance tools used to prevent a relapse of mental illness.

E-mental health support can be categorized into five groups of resources: online self-help, crisis support, medical intervention, peer-led support, and coaching ("e-Mental Health: Canada Health Infoway," n.d.). Online self-help sources allow for unguided digital interventions that help an individual learn and practice skills to manage their symptoms on their own. They also include cognitive behavioural therapy (CBT) applications like Calm, Headspace, Moodnotes, nOCD, Pacifica, PTSD Coach, BreathingRoom and TruReach. These apps teach skills, provide self-help information, and allow for symptom and thought tracking to help one manage any symptoms of anxiety, depression, Obsessive Compulsive Disorder (OCD), and Post-Traumatic Stress Disorder. Another self-guided portal called WalkAlong was developed by a group of researchers at the University of British Columbia with the support of Bell Canada's Let's Talk initiative ("About Walk Along," n.d.). It is a Canadian-based mental health resource that provides information about existing mental health care resources for friends, family, and health care professionals. It is one of many activities made to help improve the mental health of vulnerable populations through electronic resources. (Hatcher, 2014)

Interestingly, another form of online self-help technology called Electronic Problem-Solving Treatment (ePST) was developed for NASA's astronauts. It is a detailed online mobile program similar to online CBT and initially aimed to treat and manage depression in astronauts on long-duration space missions. It combines hundreds of different video clips to simulate a therapy session with an actual clinician. It includes interactive exercises such as brainstorming to help users learn skills to solve their problems. It also helps users rate their solutions to their problems in terms of advantages and disadvantages and gives them custom feedback. Users can also see reports of their progress and create action plans to prevent relapsing. This system mimics the interaction with a live clinician and is shown to be equally as effective. Although ePST was first developed for astronauts, it has been adapted for general use and is now available globally. To date, ePST users have seen a 42% decrease in depression and have reported more control over their lives. ("ePST: Problem Solving Therapy for Depression," n.d.) Research suggests that both PST and CBT can be as effective for depression as antidepressant medication with their benefits lasting long after their user stops using them as treatment (DeRubeis, 2008).

The second category of e-mental health consists of crisis support resources, which are services like phone help lines, text support, online chat support, and hotspot notifications. These offer free, immediate, and confidential one-on-one support to callers in need. They usually operate 24 hours a day, 7 days a week with paid professionals or trained volunteers as staff. They listen to the caller, offer support and advice, and try to help get the caller connected to additional help in their community if needed. (Hatcher, 2014) Examples of these lines include Kids Help Phone for Canadians aged 5-20, Good2Talk Helpline for post-secondary students, and Hope for Wellness Help Line for all Indigenous peoples across Canada.

The third group of e-mental health involves video-based and text-based counselling from clinicians and professionals, telemedicine, videoconferences, and clinical follow up and referral. These are mostly live online interactions with actual clinicians and other trained individuals, not computerized versions of them. In Halifax, the Centre for Research in Family Health started the Strongest Families Institute (SFI), which is an evidence-based, remote, and bilingual mental health service available for children, youth, and adults along with their families whenever and wherever they need it. Individuals and their families receive weekly telephone coaching from a highly trained individual who provides encouragement and problem-solving techniques. This allows users to learn the skills they need to overcome the mental health problems they face. The success rate of this service has shown to be around 85%, with less than 10% as the drop-out rate and high satisfaction reported by families overall ("Strongest Families Program," 2021). Medical and mental health intervention services like the SFI helps overcome barriers to care by delivering help and support to families right in the comfort and privacy of their homes. SFI also falls under the fifth group of e-mental health resources, which involves the use of coaching services through online therapy, videos, texts, or calls. Not only are e-coaching services convenient, but they are also personalized and effective. They provide a mentor and a guide to help individuals cope with their mental health concerns remotely, without waitlist, distance, or stigma issues.

Another group of e-mental health encompasses peer-led support initiatives. These include online monitoring, peer support apps, social media tools, chat rooms, instant messaging, and even gaming. In fact, gaming is now being used to teach cognitive behavioural skills to people in need of mental health care. While CBT techniques are usually taught by a counsellor or a psychologist or one of the aforementioned online self-help tools, they can also be taught by a game, especially when intended for teenagers. Researchers at the University of Auckland in New Zealand have created Sparx, which is a game designed to help teenagers cope with negative thoughts or feelings ("SPARX," 2009). Participants progress through different levels as part of a quest. They fight negative automatic thoughts (NATs), overcome new problems, and learn various skills at each level. In randomized controlled trials, Sparx was shown to be successful at significantly reducing depressive symptoms in 187 participants aged 12-19 (Merry et al., 2012). This makes games like Sparx a beneficial alternative to consider when treating adolescents' mental health issues through modern digital platforms.

Recent data shows that e-mental health resources are becoming increasingly important, especially in Canada. The Canadian Digital Health Survey conducted in August of 2020 showed that Canadians report a growing demand for the use of digital health services. Since 2019, access to personal health information electronically has risen up by 20%, the use of e-mental health resources has increased by 12%, and video visits with a health care provider were up by 4%. Canadians also reported a demand for services that can help them manage all aspects of their health electronically, including their mental health. They reported benefits associated with the use of virtual mental health care; 83% were satisfied with the e-mental health care they received and 72% said it helped them deal with a moment of crisis or distress that would have resulted in physical harm. Additionally, 85-86% said that e-mental health allowed them to save time and money (for transport/parking, care for dependents, time off work, time travelling, etc), 81% said that e-mental health allowed them to receive treatment faster or during after hours, and 78% said that the virtual visit helped them with the mental health concern for which they needed the appointment. ("Canadian Digital Health Survey," 2020) These recent statistics show the importance of e-mental health resources in Canada and their growing demand with the emergence of COVID-19.

Moreover, according to the MHC's E-Mental Health in Canada: Transforming the Mental Health System Using Technology document, there are two ways that technology can transform the mental health system. First is by empowering patients, and second is through more diverse platforms and resources for wider audiences. E-mental health empowers patients by making them more knowledgeable about their health conditions and by further personalizing the healthcare information and advice provided to them.

Reliable online sources allow patients to research and find information about the background of their conditions. After doing this, patients are able to reach health providers, who act as experts and as sources of information about therapeutic options. This gives patients more control over their treatment and allows them to gain reliable information to optimize their action plans. Additionally, the use of e-mental health allows for a more personalized approach to health care. With modern technology such as wearable and mobile computing and monitoring, detailed information about patients' daily habits along with a lot of physiological and behavioral data can be collected and used to help make more accurate decisions about the health care provided to patients. For instance, daily heart rate, physical activity, and sleep stage patterns can all be used to assess a mental health illness, its severity, and its treatments, which will all be specific to the patient. This empowers individuals by providing them with detailed health records, which, along with their increased knowledge about their conditions, increases their ability to articulate their needs. (Bartram, 2012)

A meta-analysis review of 13 studies with 821 participants highlights the importance of using wearable devices (such as actigraphy watches) to detect abnormal sleep and activity in patients with bipolar disorder. There were significant altered patterns of sleep in patients with bipolar disorder when compared to healthy controls (De Crescenzo, 2017). Another study assessed the impact of wearable devices and smartphones on obese participants with schizophrenia spectrum and mood disorders. Participants were given Fitbit activity tracking devices and smartphones to use for the study. Overall, participants reported that they were highly satisfied, encouraged, and motivated to reach their physical activity goals, which contributed to their overall mental and physical well-being. The study notes that lifestyle interventions aimed at promoting physical activity, like the Fitbit used, have significantly improved cardiovascular health and contributed to weight loss among people with serious mental illness in several other studies as well. (Naslund, 2016) Additionally, numerous systematic reviews and meta-analyses of randomized trials have showed the effectiveness of guided and unguided e-mental health supports for depression, anxiety, insomnia, and more (Cuijpers et al., 2010; Richards & Richardson, 2012; Andersson & Titov, 2014; Riper et al., 2014; Karyotaki et al., 2017).

Another example of the success of using mobile devices to improve the care provided to patients with mental illnesses is provided by the Maryland Psychiatric Research Center. Researchers tested the feasibility, acceptability, and preliminary efficacy of the FOCUS intervention for managing schizophrenia. FOCUS is a smartphone-based mobile intervention that offers resources to manage auditory hallucinations, social functioning, medication use, mood problems, and sleep disturbances in schizophrenic individuals. The study had 33 schizophrenic individuals use FOCUS over a 1-month period. Their paired sample t-test results showed significant reductions in psychotic symptoms, depression, and general psychopathology after the participants used FOCUS consistently for 1 month. (Ben-Zeev et al., 2017) This highlights the positive impact and potential of e-mental health resources like FOCUS and provides a method for evidence-based care and treatment to ensure consistent lifestyle management. E-mental health is overall a rapidly growing field that requires extensive and consistent improvement, support, and research. Promoting these digital solutions and innovations in e-mental health is essential for the better well-being of Canadians and others around the world, especially with the effects of the recent pandemic.

E-mental health has also been recognized for its potential applications and benefits in lower and middle-income countries. Statistics show that as much as 76–85% of people in need of treatment for mental illnesses in low- and middle-income countries do not receive any treatment at all. According to the World Health Organization, "the lack of a mental health policy, mental health programs, and mental health legislation in many countries, as well as limited resources (both financial and human), a limited infrastructure, stigma and shame are important reasons for low uptake and dissemination of mental health care" (Botlon, 2019). Therefore, digital technologies, especially those offering unguided treatments, allow these countries to overcome several of the barriers preventing them from providing mental health care. Through the internet, mental health support resources have the potential to reach millions of people quickly, efficiently, and effectively.

For instance, over 1 million people around the world use the online depression intervention 'MoodGym.' MoodGym provides anonymous, confidential, and scientifically-evaluated computerized interventions. It is an interactive and easily accessible self-help tool that helps people learn and practice skills to manage symptoms of depression and anxiety. While its effects are small and there is no therapist support, its impact on global public health can still be large, especially if it is continuously updated and improved. Other programs include 'Beating the Blues' in the United Kingdom, 'The Journal' in New Zealand, and 'MindSpot' in Australia. Several of these programs are evolving from being largely text-based, to providing treatment through videos, virtual reality, gaming, and artificial intelligence. (Hatcher, 2014) Some more free e-mental health resources in Canada include Bounceback, Wellness Together, Big White Wall, Together All, Crisis Services Canada, and AbilitiCBT. These e-mental health resources and many more can be found at ementalhealth.ca. They have numerous benefits, which are discussed in more detail in upcoming sections of this book.

The Discovery of E-mental Health

Massa Mohamed Ali

How did e-mental health become one of the most accessible and beneficial forms of health care? Where did it originate and how has it come into action?

The discovery of e-mental health came after many studies about the possible treatment options for mental illness. After mental health clinics and the internet were established around the world, e-mental health services became available. In Canada, organizations like the Canadian Mental Health Association (CMHA) and the Mental Health Commission of Canada (MHCC) were the providers of these e-mental health services after originally offering non-digital clinical care services for the mentally ill.

CMHA is one of the oldest continuing voluntary mental health organizations in Canada. It started as the Canadian National Committee for Mental Hygiene (CNCMH) in 1918 and was founded by Dr. Clarence M. Hincks and Clifford W. Beers. Before this, Beers had organized the National Committee for Mental Hygiene in 1909 in Connecticut and Hincks established a mental hygiene clinic at the Toronto Juvenile Court, which became the first in Canada. In 1920, Hincks and Beers established the International Committee for Mental Hygiene and planned for the first International Congress on Mental Hygiene, which was held in Washington in 1930. Later, the federal government created a Mental Health Grant to support all provinces in facilitating services and healthcare for the mentally ill, which helped rapidly expand the services, personnel, and research in the mental health field. Drop-in centres, a volunteer network, local branches, rehabilitation services, and visitation programs were organized across Canada making the Committee for Mental Hygiene, which was named the Canadian Mental Health Association in 1950, more successful. Many years later, ACCESS was developed, which stands for an Accessible, Continuous, Comprehensive, Effective, and Seamless mental health System. And in 1999, the official CMHA website was developed for everyone to use. ("History of CHMA," n.d.) With this website came many other websites and several services became available online, including mental health services.

According to the Mental Health Commission of Canada (MHCC) webpage, "in 2006, the Senate Standing Committee on Social Affairs, Science, and Technology completed the first-ever national study of mental health, mental illness, and addiction. The Committee's concerns [...] recommended the creation of a Mental Health Commission to provide an ongoing national focus for mental health issues. The federal government created the MHCC the following year and named the chair of the Senate Committee, the

Honourable Michael Kirby, as its first chairperson. The MHCC's first mandate (2007-2017) was to create the country's first mental health strategy" ("Who We Are," n.d.). Part of this strategy was the implementation, innovation, and continuous improvement of e-mental health services, which are now growing rapidly.

E-mental health emerged shortly after the democratization of the Internet in the 1990s. The 6th of August in 1991 was the historic day that made services like e-mental health possible. On this day, the World Wide Web became available to the public. In 1993, the World Wide Web became free for everyone to use and develop, with no fees payable (Bryant, 2021). People communicated remotely and shared their experiences with videos, images, text and sound. They exchanged information and used the new technology to their advantage. This digital revolution affected society across numerous different fields, including education, politics, journalism, entertainment, culture, health, healthcare and research. The internet provided an opportunity for all traditional in-person activities to be conducted online, including services like therapy.

The idea of online therapy was first proposed during the International Conference on Computers in 1972. Staff from Stanford and UCLA demonstrated a psychotherapy session using linked computers. They simulated a session with a licensed therapist through computer connections limited to a small network (Ainsworth, n.d.). However, even before this demonstration, another form of telehealth that was used was phone calls. Telehealth can be defined as the digitized healthcare services that are offered through a variety of modes including videoconference, internet, and telephone (Mayo Clinic Staff, 2020). Online psychotherapy initiatives were later derived from the idea of telephone psychotherapy. Although telehealth became more commonly used in the 1990s with the rise of the internet and videophone technology, it still existed in the form of telephone calls in the 1960s. By 1999 however, about 100 telehealth networks were operating with teleducation, tele-assessment, teletherapy, telemonitoring, and telesupport by many different clinicians (Green, n.d.).

Aside from the online therapy idea demonstration, some believe that the true beginning of e-mental health services is marked by the creation of Dear Uncle Ezra in 1986 (Rauch, 2017). Dear Uncle Ezra is the world's first online question and answer advice forum. It was developed by psychologist Jerry Feist and computer scientist Steve Worona at Cornell University. The platform allows questions from anyone, anywhere, and on almost any topic, with a focus on the Cornell community. Uncle Ezra was believed to be "an anonymous Cornell staffer with a mental health background" who answered the questions posed with tips and advice (Lang, 2007). Most questions addressed mental health issues and Uncle Ezra acted as a counsellor, allowing students to cope with their problems virtually and feel heard and empowered. Students asked about managing credit cards, mental and physical health, tuition, voting, housing, grades, and relationships. According to a 2007 article in the Cornell Chronicle, "over two decades Dear Uncle Ezra has posted answers to almost 20,000 queries, many from Cornell students but also from people in more than 30 countries" (Lang, 2007). Questions became archived and searchable after they were answered to help as many people as possible.

After the Dear Uncle Ezra initiative, many more electronic mental health advice services were established. For instance, therapist John Grohol developed a public mental health chat that eventually expanded to become Psych Central (Rauch, 2017). In 2004, Grohol wrote "today, e-therapy has found a niche. It is not a large niche, nor one that will attract millions of dollars in investment capital. Some small online networks of mental health practitioners continue to thrive and will likely gradually grow as more and more people learn of the benefits of online mental health services" (Rauch, 2017). Although he described the e-mental health field as a small niche at the time, it has quickly grown to become a billion dollar industry. There are now several e-mental health platforms and services available around the world. His service itself, PsychCentral, is now a popular mental health information and news website ("About PsychCentral," n.d.). Another psychologist, Leonard Holmes, contributed to the success of the e-mental health industry and developed the first fee-based mental health advice service of many more that followed. He gave participants the option of donating money to him after being offered mental health advice (Rauch, 2017).

The first online therapy that required a fee to receive online treatment from a therapist was created by Dr. David Sommers in 1995. It was also the first to provide continual dialogue and a private therapeutic relationship. Unlike the free public mental health forums known at the time, Sommers used emails and real-time private chats to provide therapy to many clients around the world. His practice more closely resembled traditional therapy because of the fee that clients paid him for his online one-on-one therapy service. Later in 1995, therapist Ed Needham became the first therapist to exclusively use chat rooms to provide therapy to clients in the United States. His service was called Cyberpsych Counselling and was also fee-based, as he charged $15 for every one hour of therapy (Rauch, 2017).

In 1997, mental health professionals established the International Society for Mental Health Online (ISMHO). Its aims included promoting and advancing online mental health treatments like online therapy. More organizations followed, focusing on the ethics and confidentiality of the e-mental health services being provided on the internet. Some of these organizations also offered training for the mental health professionals using online platforms to provide mental health care; people were trained on confidentiality, privacy and ethics matters involving online mental health services ("About ISMHO," n.d.).

Gradually, online psychotherapy practices became more popular and widespread, especially in the 2000s.

These businesses expanded to treat numerous clients at once and offer a diverse array of therapy services. Therapists started using platforms like Skype and VSee to provide video-based online therapy (Rauch, 2017). Researchers have conducted a detailed e-mental health literature review of 115 documents from 2005-2010. They found that most studies were published between 2007 and 2010, which confirmed an expected increase in the volume of literature on e-mental health over time. Of the 115 documents, 59 (51%) reported primary empirical studies, of which 25 (42%) were conducted in the United States, 13 (22%) in Australia, and 7 (12%) in the Netherlands (Lal & Adair, 2014).

According to "The History of Online Therapy" by Joseph Rauch, the first ever study about e-mental health and online therapy has not been clearly identified. However, a group of researchers at the University of Amsterdam began studying online Cognitive Behavioural Therapy (CBT) in 1996 and showed the significant positive effect of online CBT. As a result of their studies, Dutch health insurance became one of the first to start covering online CBT costs in 2005 and acknowledge the benefits of e-mental health services like online CBT. These researchers at the University of Amsterdam continued advancing their studies. Up until 2011, they had conducted nine controlled trials of online CBT for a variety of mental health disorders, among a total of 840 participants. Their overall results continue to show that online CBT is a viable and effective alternative to face-to-face treatment (Ruwaard et al., 2011).

Another study on the effects of computerized CBT was done by researchers at Columbia University in 2004. They found that participants were more satisfied with online CBT treatment than traditional therapy. Moreover, between 2006 and 2011, a study tested more than 98,000 participants before and after enrolling in the telemental health services of the U.S. Department of Veterans Affairs. The study focused on using clinic-based, high speed video conferencing as treatment. Patients received these services for an average of 182 days. This large-scale assessment of telemental health services found that the number of admissions and the days of psychiatric hospitalization decreased for both men and women by an average of about 25% after using the telemental health services provided. This study was the first to report the positive effects of teletherapy in a large population (Godleski et al., 2012).

In 2009, a smaller-scale study published on The Lancet tested 113 participants and 97 in the control group for recovery from depression in the United Kingdom. The results show that over a period of 8 months, 42% of those who received online CBT recovered from depression while only 26% of those who received traditional CBT recovered. Researchers concluded that online CBT seems to have positive effects on the treatment of depression when delivered in real time by a therapist (Kessler et al., 2009). Another study that also compared internet-based depression therapy with an equivalent face-to-face depression treatment was conducted at the University of Zurich in 2014. Researchers found that an internet-based intervention for depression is equally beneficial to regular face-to-face therapy (Wagner et al., 2014).

Moreover, in 2009, the first E-Mental Health Summit was held in the Netherlands in Amsterdam. It was organized by the Netherlands Institute of Mental Health and Addiction (Trimbos Institute) in collaboration with the International Society for Research on Internet Interventions (ISRII), VU University Amsterdam, and the University of Amsterdam. The summit included more than 500 people from over 40 countries. In total, 195 presentations were given by academics, health professionals, and policymakers, including some of the world's most respected experts on eHealth intervention evaluation and research. According to an article on the Journal of Medical Internet Research (JMIR), the "[summit's] presentations highlighted the effectiveness of Web-based treatment, new treatment developments, novel research methodologies, and the need for international collaboration" (Riper et al., 2010). The summit was a major step in the development and recognition of e-mental health services; it allowed countries to collaborate, share their research, and work on improving the online therapy services available globally.

After the summit, research and development in the e-mental health field continued to improve rapidly. In 2012, an unlimited messaging therapy smartphone application called Talkspace was launched by Oren and Roni Frank (Rauch, 2017). Although it was not the first platform to offer chat rooms for therapists and clients, it revolutionized online therapy because clients were able to send text, video, and voice messages at any time they wanted. This allowed a better overall experience for clients and gave them unlimited opportunities to get the help they needed right from their mobile smartphones. Later research also showed the positive effects of using mobile text therapy. In 2017, a Columbia University study tested for the effects of text-based online therapy. The results showed that "mobile-enabled asynchronous text therapy with a licensed therapist is an acceptable and clinically beneficial medium for individuals with various diagnoses and histories of psychological distress" (Hull & Mahan, 2017). Participants liked having the convenient access to therapy services whenever and wherever they wanted.

Since the internet became a useful resource for information, support, advice, and communication, individuals with mental health issues started increasingly using it to manage all aspects of their everyday lives. They started expecting more e-mental health options and year by year reported higher levels of technology device use. A study published on the BMC Medical Informatics and Decision Making journal also notes that "with three quarters of all lifetime cases of mental health conditions beginning by 24 years of age, and research suggesting youth view current/ traditional mental health services negatively, there [became] interest among decision-makers in harnessing eMental Health opportunities for emerging generations especially" (Wozney et al., 2017). Many countries increasingly adopted many e-mental health services. Among the first to do so was Australia. They have developed and evaluated a number of e-treatment programs and psychoeducation websites. Overall, they have been responsible for around half of the world's e-mental health programs. Over the last decade, they produced more publications on the topic than the rest of the world combined. The Australian Government was quick to acknowledge the positive research findings provide on-going financial support for the provision of these services to the public (Jorm et al., 2013).

From telephone therapy, to online forums, to online therapy, the discovery of e-mental health has benefited millions of people around the world. New e-mental health services are now continually improving and developing every day. Modern technological advancements, artificial intelligence, gaming, virtual reality are all becoming noticeable facets of online therapy. Especially with the effects of the recent pandemic, the e-mental health field is sure to become one of the most necessary, capable, and successful fields in the future.

Diffuse Impacts of Poor Mental Health

Paige Breedon

According to the Oxford dictionary, mental health is "a person's condition with regard to their psychological and emotional well-being" (Mental Health, n.d.). Therefore, the direct implications of poor mental health are psychological and emotional distress, in addition to the indirect implications of poor mental health which pertain to quality of life, social involvement, productivity, physical health, addictive behaviour, socioeconomic status, lifespan, and personal and public costs.

The diffuse nature of poor mental health is also due to its transgenerational potential, its prevalence in today's world, and its circularity. Firstly, the effects of poor mental health can transgress today's population and proceed to impact many generations to come. The transgenerational nature of mental illness is likely due to parents' psychological and epigenetic impact on their offspring (Monaco, 2021). Additionally, today's society is especially vulnerable to poor mental health considering the current COVID-19 pandemic and the consequential restrictions and lockdowns. It is also important to note that mental health is ultimately circular, as factors that contribute to poor mental health can also affect poor mental health. For that reason, mental health is a cause and effect to many problems that an individual faces. The circular nature of poor mental health, alongside transgenerational inheritance and today's pandemic, contribute to the extreme relevancy and power mental health has on today's population.

Although mental health begins with the individual, given its prevalence in today's world, the impact of poor mental health is seen throughout the community, economy, and today's youth. It is crucial to consider the implications of poor mental health and how it is so widespread. Exploring the nature of mental illness is critical in proposing relevant and effective resolutions to this budding issue.

It is essential to acknowledge that poor mental health and/or extreme consequences of emotional and psychological distress may seem innocent at first. For that reason, mental health should always be a priority to prevent many direct and indirect implications of poor mental health and to maximize one's overall quality of life. To be transparent, just because an individual does not feel mentally unhealthy does not mean they should avoid prioritizing their mental health. Mental health should always be something people consider and work toward improving.

Firstly, having poor mental health impacts one's quality of life. It can do so by a variety of means;

specifically, it can hinder one's ability to be socially and physically active; in some cases, it can be a challenge to even get out of bed. Mental illness is also something that often resides within one's psychological and emotional consciousness for many years or perhaps the entirety of one's lifetime, and therefore is always relevant and impactful for that individual.

Furthermore, a specific example of mental health's impact on an individual's productivity is its ability to limit one's success in a classroom or workplace environment. Firstly, mental health impacts one's performance in the classroom, which can inhibit students from learning and seeking higher education. This inhibition can have many other implications that can seriously alter one's life trajectory. Thus, it is essential to have conversations around student mental health to ensure today's learners, who are tomorrow's workforce members, are mentally prepared to contribute to society.

For instance, a study done in 2016 in Sweden that aimed to correlate mental health during adolescence with academic achievement later in life investigated a sample of children born in Sweden in 1990 who lived there until at least the age of 20 (Brännlund et al., 2017). Two groups of students were formed; one group was to determine the effect mental health had on completing secondary education, and the other focused on correlating mental health with grades. The experiment defined mental health problems as a student who had received at least one prescription drug. The study defined the number of years that a student was prescribed drugs for mental health as the students further descent into poor mental health. The Swedish Prescribed Drug Register provided the prescription data for the study (Brännlund et al., 2017). Firstly, students who began education in 2009 and did not graduate within three years were considered to have not completed their secondary education. Average Grade Points (AGP) was the grading scale considered for the second group of students.

On average, youth with mental-health problems had lower grades than those not prescribed drugs, and the proportion of youth with above-average grades decreased with years of treatment (Brännlund et al., 2017). Specifically at zero years of treatment, completed secondary education was just over 80% and AGP above average was 50% (Brännlund et al., 2017). After 5 years of treatment, both completed secondary education and AGP above average statistics declined to below 35% (Brännlund et al., 2017). The experiment's outcome suggested that there is an inverse and strong relationship between poor mental health and completion of secondary education (Brännlund et al., 2017). This relationship was also similar concerning grades. A limitation of the study is that the data does not reflect mentally unhealthy students who are not treated with prescribed drugs for their mental illness.

Based on the Swedish study presented, students with poor mental health are less likely to succeed in a classroom environment or academic context. It is clear that poor mental health is an extreme disadvantage to today's learners and can limit one's academic success. Considering education is often the root of future successes (i.e. career success), it is essential to prioritize student mental health to ensure a prosperous future.

Furthermore, poor mental health can affect work performance and consequently the duration and extent of employment. Poor mental health can impact an employee's ability to go into work, stay engaged, meet deadlines, and interact with colleagues and employers. Thus, people with poor mental health have a greater chance of becoming unemployed or choosing to retire early.

For instance, a 2010 Australian longitudinal population survey set to identify factors affecting retirement found that a key factor influencing retirement decisions is poor mental health. Specifically, the survey collected data from 2,803 people aged 45-75 (Olesen et al., 2011). Participants completed a Household Income and Labour Dynamics in Australia survey and had their mental health assessed according to the Mental Health Index (Olesen et al., 2011). The survey found that poor mental health was associated with higher retirement rates in men and workplace exit more generally in women (Olesen et al., 2011). Overall, poor mental and physical health was associated with early retirement based on the survey results (Olesen et al., 2011).

The Australian survey shows that mental health is associated with the age of retirement. If the trend of early retirement continues due to a mental health-related rationale, this will lead to a shrinking workforce and a consequential impact on global and economic productivity. Therefore, by prioritizing mental health in the workplace, the employee, employer, economy, and government will all benefit. Overall, poor mental health is consistent with poor academic and job performance and has the potential to lead to an uneducated and less productive population.

Additionally, mental and physical health are intimately connected. Consequently, poor mental health can lead to physical repercussions and vice versa. The relationship between physical and mental health justifies poor mental health with the potential to cause a wide range of physical problems. For instance, physical problems relating to poor mental health that are areas of interest in the field of medicine include vulnerability to disease, infection or complication after surgery, and poor fitness.

A specific 2017 study analyzed 10,653 individuals aged 50 years and older of an English population (Ohrnberger et al., 2017). The Centre for Epidemiological Studies Depression Scale and Activities of Daily Living evaluated participants' mental and physical health, respectively. The results included indirect effects explaining 10% of the effect of past mental health on physical health and 8% of the effect of past physical health on mental health (Ohrnberger et al., 2017). This study illustrates the connection between physical and mental health and how either can be a factor driving the other.

A specific example of a physical health repercussion associated with poor mental health is related to sleep. A longitudinal study of Japanese junior high school students was completed in the early 2000s to examine the relationship between sleep and mental health status (Kaneita et al., 2009). Specifically, 698 subjects completed a baseline survey in 2004 and 516 subjects returned for the follow-up survey in 2006 (Kaneita et al., 2009).The Pittsburgh Sleep Quality Index was used to determine sleep quality and disturbances, and the Japanese version of the 12-item General Health Questionnaire allowed for the calculation of a score reflective of the student's mental health. The difference from 2004 to 2006 showed an increase in sleep disturbances from 39.5% to 48.1% (Kaneita et al., 2009).This increase was consistent with an increase in the prevalence of poor mental health, which increased from 38.2% to 44.4% (Kaneita et al., 2009). The study clearly illustrates a relationship between sleep and mental health: specifically, lack of sleep can affect one's mental health, and mental health can affect one's quality and duration of sleep. Sleep is just one example of a physical implication of poor mental health.

Also, poor mental health is often a contributor to addiction. Addictions due to mental illness can include but are not limited to alcohol and drugs. For instance, a study including 1254 first-year university students from a mid-sized private university in northeastern United

States living on campus had participants complete an online survey (Kenney et al., 2018). Students were asked questions regarding alcohol use and mental health and the results ultimately concluded that higher anxiety and depression lead to greater consumption of alcoholic beverages (Kenney et al., 2018). This study demonstrates that poor mental health makes students more at risk of heavy drinking or susceptible to these types of behaviour. Clearly, a relationship exists between addictive behaviour and poor mental health.

Moreover, poor mental health can also have an impact on one's socioeconomic status and contributions to society. As previously mentioned, poor mental health can decrease productivity and job performance and, therefore, can result in unemployment. Unemployment can ultimately lead to homelessness, poverty, and a state where the individual is no longer contributing to society. These effects are hard to reverse and tend to worsen one's mental health, thus maintaining the characteristic circularity of the problem.

Another repercussion of being a victim of mental illness is the chance of being discriminated against due to one's mental illness or mental health-related problems. For instance, a study published in 2018 looked at 301 unemployed individuals recruited from unemployment agencies in Southern Germany with mental health issues to examine the discrimination they may have experienced on both the level of unemployment and poor mental health (Staiger et al., 2018). Group participants who experienced both levels of discrimination reported lower job search self-efficacy, more perceived stigma-related barriers to care, and more need for treatment than participants who felt mainly discriminated against due to unemployment (Staiger et al., 2018). This study concluded that experiencing discrimination due to mental illness and/or unemployment can affect job search and help-seeking among this demographic of individuals. Awareness about the stigma surrounding mental illness and unemployment needs to continue to contribute to a mentally healthy tomorrow.

The most invaluable cost of poor mental health is self-harm and suicide. The effects are unimaginably painful for the family members left behind and can proceed to emotionally burden them for many years if not the complete duration of their lifetime. A study carried out 3275 psychological autopsies of people who have committed suicide. The results showed that 87.3% had been diagnosed with a mental disorder prior to death (Arsenault-Lapierre et al., 2004). More specifically, 43.2% of suicide cases were diagnosed with affective disorders (including depressive and bipolar disorders) and 25.7% with other substance problems (Arsenault-Lapierre et al., 2004). Also, 16.2% of people had personality disorders that have affected their mental health with some margin for error (Arsenault-Lapierre et al., 2004). This relationship shows just how extreme the effects of poor mental health can be and also emphasizes the importance of prioritizing mental health awareness and resources for those who need help.

Furthermore, poor mental health comes at a cost for the inflicted, the government, the taxpayer, and the employer. For the individual specifically, there are both direct and indirect costs associated with poor mental health. Directly, people who have mental illness depending on the health care infrastructure of their country may have costs associated with treatment, medication, and hospitalization. Also, indirectly because of one's mental illness, there is a cost associated with loss of productivity and, perhaps in the most extreme cases, life. In the United States alone, mental health disorders cost nearly $193 billion in lost earnings each year (Khushalani et al., 2018). This is a staggering statistic and another reason to prioritize mental health.

Also, the cost of healthcare associated with mental health for a country can be overwhelming. In the United States, the cost of annual mental health care spending is approximately $201 billion (Khushalani et al., 2018). This cost justifies just how important it is to prioritize mental health and how poor mental health can have severe consequences not only for the individual but for the economy, country, and the globe. Although the severity of mental health costs may differ between countries, no country will remain unscathed from poor mental health effects, whether those effects are primarily economic or otherwise.

After carefully considering the immense impact mental health can have on an individual and economy, it is vital to consider why mental illness is so widespread and influential. Poor mental health is a condition that is both a cause and effect of many other problems. For that reason, it is circular, and the circularity of mental health makes resolving and preventing transgenerational mental illness very challenging. Specifically, parental influences drive the transgenerational nature of mental illness. Firstly, the values and mentality parents hold that are conducive to their poor mental health can be easily passed on to their offspring through how they teach their children and the behaviours that their children observe and pick up.

Moreover, changes to one's germline epigenome due to lifestyle and environmental factors can be passed onto offspring, resulting in mental illness progressing to future generations (Monaco, 2021). According to the National Human Genome Research Institute, Epigenetics is "an emerging field of science that studies the heritable changes caused by the activation and deactivation of genes without any change in the underlying DNA sequence of the organism" (Epigenetics, n.d.). Various environmental and lifestyle factors can change the epigenetic pattern of an individual and, therefore, allow for transgenerational inheritance (Monaco, 2021). Based on this information, epigenetics is a mechanism by which poor mental health can impact future generations, and the further exploration of this field can help work toward a mentally healthy tomorrow. Overall, mental illness is widespread due to its intimate connection with many other facets of health and its ability to operate in a cycle. In order to combat poor mental health, therefore, approaches need to consider the circular nature in which mental health operates and trends in transgenerational inheritance.

In conclusion, poor mental health has immense effects and tenaciously repeats itself. Poor mental health starts with challenging an individual's emotional, social, and physical health and proceeds to affect the greater public through the economy. Poor mental health is directly related to a less productive society inside the classroom and workplace as well as a more socially distant society. Being mentally unhealthy also makes an individual more susceptible to physical health implications such as problems with quality and duration of sleep. Poor mental health is often the root of many addictions, and those addictions seem to worsen one's mental health further, thus continuing the vicious cycle of mental illness. Mental illness also can impact one's socioeconomic status and contributions to society. Specifically, mental illness can impact one's ability to obtain and maintain quality employment and stay above the poverty line. Being mentally handicapped can also put one into a category where they are vulnerable to discrimination which keeps one in a difficult position to find work and receive proper help and treatment. In the most extreme and devastating cases, poor mental health can lead to self-harm and/or suicide. This cost is exceptionally relevant and prevalent in today's society and affects many loved ones left behind. The direct and indirect financial cost of mental illness is also immense. However, the financial burden also affects those not directly impacted by mental illnesses as community members and taxpayers. Employers of people with poor mental health also have to pay in the form of loss of productivity and direct costs such as sick days.

Additionally, the generational prevalence and circularity of mental health characterize its diffuse nature. Specifically, parental influences such as behaviour, epigenetics, and the environment they create for their offspring can all lead to poor mental health, hindering future generations. Mental health is not linear; it is circular in the sense that it is a cause and effect, and therefore if one is mentally unhealthy, they will be affected by consequences that will continue to worsen their mental health. The transgenerational potential and circular nature of mental health are why solutions are frequently ineffective and are therefore where time should be invested to lead to a better tomorrow.

Especially in today's world, where the COVID-19 pandemic is quite restricting and socially isolating, mental health is more important than ever. Considering its prevalence, immense effects, and widespread capability, it is a significant priority to understand, educate, and prioritize better mental health to lead to a more prosperous and productive future. Perhaps the solution, especially in today's socially distant world, lies in the use of electronic mental health resources to help those with poor mental health, as well as the general public, better understand and appreciate the importance of prioritizing mental health.

Importance of E-mental Health in Today's Society

Hafsa Binte Younus

As seen in the previous chapter, poor mental health has a diffuse nature as it immensely impacts the life of the individual who suffers and the lives of those around them. Especially in today's society, where the COVID-19 pandemic has also had a major impact on almost every aspect of life and has spread the feeling of uncertainty and fear throughout the entire nation. Since the start of COVID-19, the need for mental health services has increased more than ever before. COVID-19 has forced human civilization to completely change the lifestyle they were used to living and adapt to a new normal inducing a lot of anxiety. This chapter will focus on e-mental health and its importance today.

Mental Health in Today's Society due to COVID-19

Today, the uncertainty around COVID-19 is impacting everyone's habits and overall style of living with social distancing, wearing masks, using sanitizers, and regularly washing hands becoming the new norm. Everyone is living with a sense of uncertainty, wanting answers to all the unknowns. Although

41

at first sight, the COVID-19 pandemic, an acute respiratory syndrome outbreak, is a crisis that impacts an individual's physical health, on closer inspection it is evident that it has negatively impacted people's mental health too. The COVID-19 pandemic has posed new threats to families through social isolation due to physical distancing measures, school/childcare closures, financial and employment insecurity, housing instability, and changes to health and social care access. The trauma associated with the loss caused by COVID-19 and stress associated with government-imposed lockdowns/stay-at-home orders and severe social distancing has affected almost all age groups; whether it be from school-going children to young-university students or working-class individuals to retired senior citizens (Hossain et al., 2020).

A recent review has found that quarantine and similar prevention strategies can result in the manifestation of depression, anxiety disorders, mood disorders, posttraumatic stress symptoms, sleep disorders, panic, stigmatization, low self-esteem, and lack of self-control in isolated individuals (Hossain et al., 2020). Another review has shown that stressors caused by COVID-19 (i.e. prolonged quarantine, constant fear of infection, boredom, inadequate knowledge and supplies, financial loss, and stigma) can result in long-lasting posttraumatic stress symptoms, confusion, and anger within the population (Hossain et al., 2020).

Moreover, according to Statistics Canada's Survey on COVID-19 and Mental Health, impacts of the pandemic such as increased social isolation, job and income loss, and difficulties meeting financial obligations could negatively influence mental health (Statistics Canada, 2021). It states that although symptoms such as changes in behavior, thoughts, and feelings are a normal response to stressful situations, experiencing these symptoms constantly and excessively can undermine one's well-being and quality of life (Statistics Canada, 2021). Findings from the survey indicated that almost one in five (21%) of Canadian adults aged 18 and older screened positive for at least of the following three mental disorders: 1. major depressive disorder (MDD); 2. generalized anxiety disorder (GAD); 3. post-traumatic stress disorder (PTSD) (Statistics Canada, 2021). Of those who were screened positive for any of the three disorders, about 68% reported that their mental health had worsened due to the COVID-19 pandemic. Therefore, providing proper mental health support is crucial (Statistics Canada, 2021). Moreover, even though mental health was a huge concern before the pandemic, it has worsened after the pandemic hit with almost 68% of Canadians reporting good mental health in 2019 (before pandemic) down to only 55% of Canadians reporting good mental health by July 2020 (during pandemic) (Statistics Canada, 2020).

The pandemic has also affected the mental health of many parents as well. Since the start of the pandemic and lockdowns, many parents have experienced increased pressures such as erosions to social support, the burden of becoming the sole supervisor to their children, having increased responsibility of providing education for their children, and experiencing heightened financial and emotional stress (Gadermann et al., 2021). A study done by Gadermann et al. which examined the impact of COVID-19 on family mental health in Canada showed that COVID-19 has worsened the mental health of around 44.3% of parents with children younger than 18 years old living at home and 35.6% of respondents without children younger than 18 years old living at home (Gadermann et al., 2021). Moreover, parents compared to the rest of the sample also reported increased alcohol consumption, suicidal thoughts/feelings, and stress about being safe from physical/emotional domestic violence (Gadermann et al., 2021). Not only that, around 24.8% of parents reported that their children's mental health had also worsened since the beginning of the pandemic and that the pandemic had also resulted in them having more frequent negative interactions with their children (Gadermann et al., 2021).

COVID-19 has not only impacted the mental health of adults but has also significantly impacted the lives and mental health of children and youth too. For example, before COVID-19 and lockdown, children and adolescents predominantly learned through one-to-one interactions with their mentors and peers (Singh et al., 2020). However, the unfortunate nationwide closure of schools, colleges, and universities has negatively impacted almost 91% of the world's student population (Singh et al., 2020). Due to COVID-19, children and youth have now suddenly lost access to many of the activities, such as school, extracurricular activities, social interactions, and physical activity, that previously provided structure, meaning, rhythm, and routine to their lives (Singh et al., 2020). The home confinement of children and adolescents has resulted in the disruption of their education along with their physical and social lives (Singh et al., 2020). Children and youth are experiencing way more boredom and are experiencing a lack of innovative ideas for engaging in various academic and extracurricular activities as almost all extracurriculars have either halted or transitioned to the online platform due to lockdowns (Singh et al., 2020). This is also resulting in children becoming a lot more clingier, attention-seeking, and dependent on parents (Singh et al., 2020). Moreover, studies have also found that older adolescents and youth have an increased level of anxiousness regarding examination cancellation and overall, all the academic events (Singh et al., 2020). Over time, this isolation, lack of social support, and anxiousness may result in depressive symptoms in the children and youth. This social withdrawal, loneliness, and hopelessness may result in them developing poor mental health (Singh et al., 2020).

These are just a few examples of how COVID-19 has impacted the lives and mental health of people globally and it can be understood that today the need for mental health awareness and services has increased dramatically as everyone is living in fear and uncertainty associated with COVID-19. Moreover, in the previous chapter, it was understood that the impact of poor mental health can last over generations. Therefore, it is extremely important to address this issue and provide proper interventions and services to people. Now the concern is how can the people's mental health be addressed and how can the mental health services be provided during lockdowns and while taking full precautions and ensuring everyone's safety. This is where e-mental health becomes very important.

Technology and E-mental Health

Today, technology is an integral part of the world and people's daily routine. It has allowed us to access almost the entire world and resources at our fingertips. It has affected the way individuals communicate, learn, and think. It allows people living on opposite sides of the world to interact daily and easily. Technology and the innovative applications associated with it have brought many new methods of electronic communication such as video conferencing, chats, emails, posts, and so on. This advancement allows people to stay in touch and communicate while keeping everyone safe and healthy. Especially during the COVID-19 pandemic, the internet and technology are something that has allowed people to stay connected and continue with their lives. When everything is in lockdown and people are forced to isolate themselves due to the COVID-19 pandemic, the use of technology has increased immensely. The lockdown has resulted in most people relying on the internet and internet-based services to communicate, interact, and continue with their educational, and employment responsibilities from home (De' et al., 2020). The usage of internet services has risen from being 40% to 100%, compared to pre-lockdown levels (De' et al., 2020). Especially video-conferencing services such as Zoom have experienced a ten times increase in usage as almost all major forms of professional communications take place on that platform (De' et al., 2020).

The health industry has also adapted to the technological advancements and has developed many innovative apps, such as calorie counters, heart rate modulators, and other telehealth apps, through which people can access health care services more easily and at any time of the day (Monaghesh & Hajizadeh, 2020). Today, the health care system has significantly adapted to the online mode of providing health care services (telehealth) (Monaghesh & Hajizadeh, 2020). A systematic review study showed that currently, healthcare providers and patients who are self-isolating are majorly relying on telehealth to ensure the minimization of the risk of COVID-19 transmission (Monaghesh & Hajizadeh, 2020). This solution potentially prevents any sort of direct physical contact between people, while it provides continuous accessible health care to the community (Monaghesh & Hajizadeh, 2020). The use of telehealth reduces morbidity and mortality in COVID-19 outbreaks (Monaghesh & Hajizadeh, 2020). Therefore, telehealth has become an important tool in caring services while keeping patients and health providers safe during the COVID-19 outbreak (Monaghesh & Hajizadeh, 2020).

Just like telehealth, providing online mental health services is also extremely important. As previously mentioned, the need for diagnosis, care, treatment, and other services associated with mental health have greatly increased since the start of the COVID-19 pandemic and have become a huge concern in today's society. Although the need for mental health services in Canada and across the world is significant, the traditional mental health delivery model which requires people to access the services in person is not sufficient to provide services to everyone, especially during the COVID-19 pandemic where everyone is forced to social distance and isolate (Moock, 2014). Therefore, innovative ideas such as pairing technology and mental health services have found their place today to provide essential mental health services to people and improve the current scenario of high demand and limited access to mental health services. This use of information and communication technology related to the internet to provide mental health services is known as e-mental health (Moock, 2014). E-mental services are internet-based interventions that can encompass a variety of modalities including videoconferencing, computer games, web-based therapy, text messages, virtual reality, and many more (Moock, 2014). It can also include real-time interaction with trained clinicians as well as mental health applications and links on mobile phones, peer support services, and computer-based programs (Moock, 2014). According to the National Health Service (NHS) Network of the NHS Confederation, e-mental health is the use of information and communication technologies to support and improve mental health, including the use of online resources, social media, and smartphone applications (Moock, 2014). More information about what exactly e-mental health is will be provided in the following chapters.

Although e-mental health was launched a long time ago (i.e. by around 2005 in Canada) (Jeong et al., 2019), the COVID-19 crisis today has highlighted the important role of telehealth and digital tools to provide care in times of need (Torous et al., 2020). After being forced for the first time to use these tools to connect and provide services when face-to-face connections are impossible, both the clinicians and patients are now realizing the full potential of these telehealth services (Torous et al., 2020). Seeing today's situation, e-mental health (Telehealth) seems the right mode of delivery for mental health care.

Importance of E-mental Health

First of all, e-mental health presents patients with a convenient and flexible option to freely decide and choose where their treatment will take place (The Royal Australian College of General Practitioners, 2015). They do not have to specially go out to be able to access services. This way, e-mental health removes the barriers such as the barrier of social distancing and lockdowns and allows people to access care safely. There is also strong evidence that supports that e-mental health interventions successfully help people manage mild to moderate depression and anxiety (The Royal Australian College of General Practitioners, 2015); two of the most common mental health issues

(Dobson et al., 2020.). As mentioned earlier, anxiety and depression are also two of the most common mental health issues associated with the COVID-19 pandemic. E-mental health resources and services also allow people to access and review educational material as often as they like and increase their knowledge about mental health and how to cope with it (The Royal Australian College of General Practitioners, 2015). They can also access and proceed with the services they need at their own pace without the constant pressure of being accountable to someone (The Royal Australian College of General Practitioners, 2015). E-mental health is a cost-effective method that provides more equitable access to care as it is typically lower in cost (The Royal Australian College of General Practitioners, 2015). Other than the cost of the internet plan and device that the patient decides to use to access the services, e-mental health services such as peer support, online forums, educational resources suggested therapies are often free of cost. This way, more people (including people with low incomes) would be able to afford the services and benefit from them without being financially burdened. It would also increase mental health service accessibility and allow residents of rural areas, where face-to-face mental health services are extremely rare and hard to find, to access internet-delivered services and education and be able to benefit from them (The Royal Australian College of General Practitioners, 2015). Thus, the barriers that are associated with geographic isolation, travel, and distance would be addressed. Additionally, patients who tend to avoid the traditional mental health services due to feelings of shame, embarrassment, stigma, or concerns about confidentiality, would also easily be able to access these services without the fear of being judged and known by people (The Royal Australian College of General Practitioners, 2015). Moreover, certain services such as peer-to-peer support and other online resources can be accessed using a variety of devices such as phones, tablets, and laptops, 24/7. Moreover, since more people would be able to access treatment using online platforms and helplines, the waiting time before one can access help and services is also reduced allowing people to access the services immediately. This would allow the physician to focus more on complicated and urgent cases. Moreover, e-mental health resources can also be used to educate and spread awareness about mental health. Lastly and most importantly, e-mental health would also allow people to connect and have a sense of community. This is extremely important especially during such an unfortunate time of the COVID-19 crisis as being able to connect with others would help reduce people's sense of loneliness which in turn would improve their mental health.

Conclusion

To conclude, according to current situations, e-mental health seems to be extremely important and the right solution towards improving accessibility of and promoting mental health services in today's society. E-mental health tools have the potential to improve the quality as well as increase access to mental health care services. However, there are many benefits, drawbacks, and many other concerns such as safety, reliability, confidentiality, etc. that are associated with e-mental health. All of these topics will be discussed in future chapters. In the next chapter, the topic "what exactly is e-mental health?" will be explored.

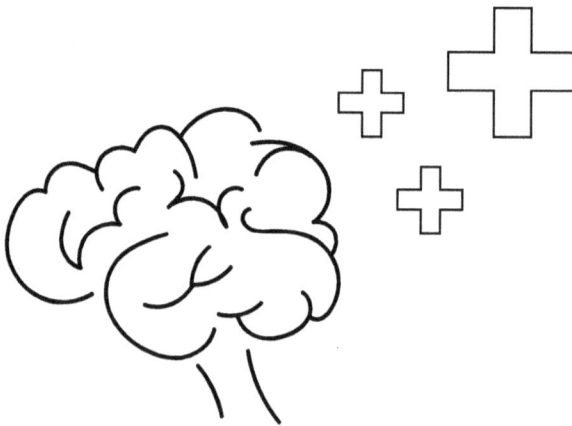

What is E-mental health?

Jannat Irfan

According to the World Health Organization (2004) and Galderisi et al. (2015), mental health is a "state of well-being in which the individual realizes his or her abilities, can cope with the normal stresses of life, can work productively and fruitfully, and is able to make a contribution to his or her community" (World Health Organization, 2004; Galderisi et al., 2015). However, during these tough times of COVID-19, many people are struggling mentally and are developing mental illnesses. Findings from a 2020 Statistics Canada survey on mental health during COVID-19 shows that one in five (21%) Canadian adults aged 18 and older are screened positive for at least one mental illness or mental disorder (Statistics Canada, 2020). The survey assessed the following mental disorders: major depressive disorder, anxiety disorder and post-traumatic disorder (Statistics Canada, 2020). These findings show that Canadians are struggling with their mental health due to the current situation with COVID-19 as well as other personal issues and problems that they were experiencing before COVID-19 and are in need of attention. The question is where can these people receive help from?

As technology advances, the ways people can be treated both physically and mentally have advanced too. In Canada, the use of technology to control, detect, screen, or treat a patient is very common (Hatcher et al., 2014). Almost all Canadians use technology such as their smartphones, computers and the internet on a daily basis for various purposes such as transactions, communicating with other people through social media and emails, and handling their finances. Technology is very trusted in our society but why is it not trusted for mental health services online? One of the reasons for this mistrust in people can be the limitations such as regional, profession, and resources (Hatcher et al., 2014). However, this is slowly changing and the way we use technology is transforming in new ways as the use of technology becomes more popular (Hatcher et al., 2014). A lot of people use the internet to get both physical and mental health services because of multiple benefits of telehealth and e-mental health services that will be discussed later in this chapter.

E-mental health is an abbreviation for electronic mental health. E-mental health is the use of mental health services and information that are delivered to people using the internet and technology (Mucic et al., 2016). It is essentially the use of telecommunication and information technologies to deliver mental health services at a distance (Mucic et al., 2016). E-mental health is delivered to patients in the form of video capture of a patient's history and forwarding it to a psychiatrist, patients email, online mental health services such as kids help phone, and other internet-based methods. Mohr et al (2013) defines e-mental health as a type of technology that includes telephone and videoconferencing services, web-based interventions which are known as internet interventions, interventions using mobile phones, integration of sensors for patient monitoring, social media, visual reality, and games (Hatcher et al., 2014).

As discussed earlier, e-mental health especially these days is a very popular option for people in Canada as well as people all around the world due to the tough situation of COVID-19 the world is going through right now. COVID-19 has impacted people's lives a lot in terms of education, work, and personal life. It is causing people to fear and worry for their health and the health of their loved ones as they are at high risk of developing mental illnesses. Ofcourse, e-mental health did exist before COVID-19 too and many people used it and are still using it because of how accessible it is to every population. To cope with their mental illness, many people use the internet in hopes to have good mental health by participating in various programs or contacting online mental health services. They tend to use e-mental health services because e-mental provides patients with the opportunity to be empowered by the provisions of health information so that when the health providers are no longer the sole holders of knowledge regarding the illness and disease (Hatcher et al., 2014). According to Cotton et al (2013), "The greater use of the information and the technology could help people address resource challenges as well as it has the potential to support cultural transformation and move towards a social model of health, by empowering service users to exercise greater choice and control and to manage their conditions more effectively." This allows the patients to have more control and know more about their health conditions and hence be more aware of their needs and how to fulfill those needs whereas their healthcare providers act as both experts and the person whom the patients can ask to receive more information about the therapeutic options (Hatcher et al., 2014). Another reason that people levitate towards receiving e-mental health services is that it does not cost much and it is very accessible to all general populations even those living in rural areas. It does not have as many limitations to it as in-person mental health services do.

Moreover, on the internet, many non-profit e-mental health organizations can provide mental health services to people as well as people can meet peers on the internet and get the support they need. It has been found that the role of peer support in terms of e-mental health is seen as very valuable as peer support helps and support the people with lived experience of mental illness can give to another person (CMHA National, 2019). Peer supporters can share their knowledge and experiences with the person who is struggling mentally and provide the support that a counsellor or a therapist can not (CMHA National., 2019). Peer support is basically the opportunity to look for and receive support from others who have previously faced similar problems and asking them for advice or just talking to them (Hatcher et al., 2014). Peer support is a very famous option for people who use e-mental health services as it is easier to find a peer with similar experiences online than in-person due to different time zones and living in different cities or countries. There are multiple advantages of doing peer support online such as the opportunity to talk to many people with the same experience as you at the same time in group chats and give each other advice. An example of peer support through social media and other technologies is Big White Wall (http://www.bigwhitewall.com) which is an online e-mental health service where the users are anonymous and are looking for help to cope with their mental illness or psychological distress (Hatcher et al., 2014). Big White Wall also provides peer-to-peer support e-mental health services which are called Togetherhall which is accessible to anyone who has a phone or a computer. In addition, Big White wall provides e-mental health services to people aged from 16+ 24/7 and users can immediately be able to talk to trained Big White Wall staff whose job is to make sure the community is safe and support is provided to everyone who is struggling (https://cmhact.ca/news/new-online-peer-support-and-self-management-tool-free-in-ontario). Furthermore, the clients who use Big White wall also have access to the online guided courses which they can take with users who are in the same situation as them and have the same concerns. By taking these courses together on various topics can lead them to heal together (https://cmhact.ca/news/new-online-peer-support-and-self-management-tool-free-in-ontario). This anonymous e-mental health service allows the users to be anonymous and talk about their concerns without worrying about their privacy and without fearing that someone they know might find out about their mental illness. Another example is Mindyourmind (http://www.mindyourmind.ca) which is also an e-mental health support service for the youth and adults in Ontario, Canada. The forum mainly uses youth networks to yield a platform for youth where they can talk about their mental health, their mental health illness, look for advice, and lastly support the creation of resources for youth and adults with mental illness (Hatcher et al., 2014). Many online mental health services provide additional peer support as discussed before. The peer supporter either calls or messages via email with the other person and shares coping stories with the other person to help them navigate the mental health system, encourage, inspire, and support them. Moreover, a peer supporter can be a coach too and there is increasing evidence that the presence of a coach, who may not or maybe a clinician can improve the outcomes of a person struggling with mental illness using the internet or computerized resources (Hatcher et al., 2014). The mental health commission (Hatcher et al., 2014) stated that "where access to psychological treatments is difficult, the potential for computerized therapies to provide treatments without waiting lists and at a time and place of patients' choosing is obvious." This again indicates that e-mental health services are more accessible to people compared to in-person mental health services. Moreover, it has been found that computerized therapies via phone and email save more time, for both the person receiving therapy and the person providing therapy service and hence freeing up professionals to spend more time with more severe cases (Hatcher et al., 2014). In addition, as stated earlier, computerized therapies are now shifting onto phones and multiple mental health apps can be found for free (Hatcher et al., 2014). Everyone these days have at least one technology device and many people under the age of 16 use technology as well to connect with friends. Hence, there is an e-mental health service in Canada that is specifically targeted for populations who are not adults. This e-mental health service is known as the Kids Help Phone and people who require mental support can reach out to Kids helps phone via text message, phone call, Facebook messenger, or a live chat. Kids Help Phone offers counselling to Canadians who are between the ages of five to twenty and this service is available 24/7 and all days of the year (Hatcher et al., 2014). Kids Help Phone also has another service named As Us Online which lets users express their feelings and mental state and ask questions anonymously. The Kids Help Phone Staff and volunteers would then reply to the users' posts asynchronously. The posts made by users can be viewed by thousands of youth that visit the Ask Us online platform and they can gain information regarding their mental illness without posting. Kids Help Phone has been known to be a very efficient e-mental health service as it has been found during an evaluation that users who use the Kids Help Phone e-mental health services experience significant results over key clinical indicators such as decreased mental distress and an increase in confidence and clarity (Hatcher et al., 2014). Moreover, Kids Help Phone is free and also has a free app that can be downloaded on a phone and the app has a recorder that includes features such as feeling logs, stress busters, advice and tips, jokes, inspirational quotes, resources around me tool, and lastly connecting with a counsellor tool through live chat or phone call (Hatcher et al., 2014). Gaming is also another e-mental health service that is provided for people who are not comfortable talking to someone whether it be via technology or in-person. Gaming is a good way to learn and teach cognitive behavioural skills to people who experience mental health illnesses and problems (Hatcher et al., 2014). An example would be a game known as Sparx (http://www.sparx.org.nz) which is based upon an imaginary island where the participants who are playing the game have a battle with negative automatic thoughts during the battle to progress in the game (Hatcher et al., 2014). The game's main audiences are youth and it has been shown that games that promote e-mental health services can be equally effective in treating mild to moderate depression through a randomized controlled trial study (Hatcher et al., 2014).

As discussed earlier, the internet is frequently used for mental health services in Canada and all around the world. In total there are 25.5 million Canadian internet users, and every one of them is online every day especially the youth (Hatcher et al., 2014). It has been said that the youth is most attracted by e-mental health services because it is very accessible to them and mental health is becoming less of a taboo in the 21st century. Moreover, e-mental health is a great way to help young males who are struggling with their mental health as males are the most reluctant ones to get mental health services (Ybarra & Eaton, 2005; Rickwood, Deane, & Wilson, 2007; Hatcher et al., 2014). In another study on older youth, it was found out that 31% of university students searched the internet for mental health information and services (Horgan & Sweeney, 2010). Hence, these studies above show that e-mental health heavily attracts the youth since they are the ones who use devices such as phones the most.

Since devices with the internet are very common in the world, people from all ethnicities can access them. For example, in Canada, there are various peer support networks, computerized interventions, and therapies for First Nations, Inuit, and Metis populations (Hatcher et al., 2014). Since having a proper internet connection and having access to broadband capacity can be challenging sometimes especially for communities living in rural and remote areas, workstations are being made which are based on the patient's computers and slowly various software interventions are bringing next generation e-mental health services to the rural and remote population (Hatcher et al., 2014).

Overall, e-mental health services are known to improve the quality, efficiency, and inequity of mental health services that are provided in Canada (Hatcher et al., 2014). From the perspective of a user, e-mental health services are very convenient and can provide mental health services for any age group and at any time without any wait (Hatcher et al., 2014). Moreover, e-mental health services have been proven to be just as effective as in-person mental health services and reliable evidence from various studies indicates that e-mental health interventions do more good than harm (Hatcher et al., 2014). The National Institute for Clinical Excellence recommends e-mental health services for mild to moderate depression as well as the systematic reviews for the computerized treatments of mental health illness have demonstrated them to be more effective than no treatment at all (Hatcher et al., 2014). In addition, one of the biggest advantages of e-mental health services is that these services can be implemented with high fidelity and can be easily personalized for a user hence which leads to better outcomes and high efficacy for patients overcoming their mental illness and mental problem challenges (Hatcher et al., 2014). This shows that e-mental health services can be very user-friendly and may be able to make a user comfortable while using the service (Hatcher et al., 2014).

In conclusion, the field of technology and e-mental health are advancing and changing quickly for a better future. E-mental health is a great way for people to find the immediate help and attention that they deserve. Mental illnesses are a real thing and anyone can be affected by them. E-mental health plays a very strong role in promoting mental health awareness and useful resources as well as helping people overcome their mental illness through various e-mental health services.

Benefits and Possible Contraindications of E-mental Health

Abeer Ansari

People from all parts of the world and socioeconomic backgrounds can struggle with their mental health on any given occasion. Poor mental health and mental disorders are prevalent in almost every industrialized country and affects people of all ages and genders (Moock, 2014). While there is still stigma surrounding the topic of mental health struggles, society has advanced in mental health advocacy and has started revolutionizing the mental health landscape in various communities. This has led to the success of various psychological interventions such as group therapies, psychotherapy, couples therapy, cognitive behaviour therapy, as well as the combination of therapy and medications. While people have started to accept the idea of psychological treatments and many around the world have benefitted from these interventions, the lack of access to mental health services remains a huge problem when it comes to accessing quality healthcare (Moock, 2014). Individuals should have access to unrestricted mental health services in order for communities to progress and promote mental well-being. The quality of the treatment for mental disorders and poor mental health is continuously evolving for the better with new expertise in the field. However, this advancement is not taking place in every region of the world and hence there are individuals who do not have access to quality medical care. This gap in the healthcare system can be addressed by implementing e-mental health services which are essentially mental health treatment delivered via the Internet (Moock, 2014). Moreover, it's also important to examine how COVID-19 has impacted the access to mental health services. Perhaps this is a time to navigate and implement the use of e-mental health to deliver effective treatment so people all around the world who are being impacted by the psychological effects of COVID-19 can access the support they need (Situmorang, 2020). The internet has become an integral part of our lives as it is a source of communication, education and entertainment. Essentially, e-mental health includes mental health apps and web pages that offer educational tools and information about mental health, peer support groups, virtual interventional programs and sessions with clinicians. However, while the use of e-mental health will bring numerous benefits, the internet is rapidly evolving and thus new challenges may arise with using technology to deliver mental health care (Wise et al, 2016). Hence, this chapter will provide an in depth review of the benefits and possible contraindication of e-mental health.

E-mental health offers a wide range of benefits that have the potential to positively impact not only the consumers of those services but also the economy as it happens to be a cost-effective way of delivering mental health resources (Moock, 2014). As defined in previous chapters, e-mental health refers to treatment and intervention based services, educational resources and really any virtual tool related to mental health. These benefits will be discussed in detail in the following paragraphs. E-mental health services that are centered towards patient care, such as having online appointments with a clinician and accessing therapy via virtual platforms, patients do not have to worry about the long wait times which helps in getting an early diagnosis as well as an early intervention and treatment plan. This prevents patients from suffering with untreated illnesses for a prolonged period of time and thus promotes a progressive solution for a mentally healthy community (Moock, 2014).

Researchers have analyzed data from the mental health services data set as well as the Health of the Nation Outcome Scale to understand the relationship between wait times of mental health services and patient's health outcomes (Reichert, 2018). An analysis of this data illustrates that longer wait times for treatment has resulted in poor mental health outcomes. The effects are extremely detrimental when the wait times range between 3 months to 12 months (Reichert, 2018). Therefore, the fact that e-mental health services help patients avoid the long wait times before accessing treatment is a huge achievement in terms of delivering quality care and increasing treatment efficacy. E-mental health also increases efficiency by allowing people to access information online without having to travel long distances or spend large amounts of money (Moock,

2014). The easy and efficient access to information also simplifies the entire process of trial and error during which a patient tries out different resources to figure out which one works best for them. E-mental health services such as tele-therapy promotes flexibility for both the patient and the physician by allowing them to schedule appointments from the comfort of their homes. In addition to efficiency, e-mental health services also provide accessibility to a wider range of population that was otherwise neglected as they lacked accessible mental health care. This serves to bridge the gap between people of different cultures, races and socioeconomic backgrounds and hence promotes equity in healthcare (Moock, 2014). Besides the patient centered e-mental health treatments and interventions, there are also great educational tools available virtually which makes information related to mental health and mental illness readily available to everyone around the world with access to technology. This worldwide access to information allows people to be more self aware and results in increased mental health literacy. The stigma surrounding mental health is still very prevalent in all communities and cultures, however, access to educational materials will enable health practitioners and instructors to initiate conversations around mental health and explore different resources that can enhance their learning. In some communities and cultures, the stigma is much more prevalent than in others and different cultural groups perceive mental health struggles in unique ways which impacts the type of treatments and resources they wish to reach out to (Reichert, 2018). Immigrant mental health is one prime example of how moving countries and settling into a new culture can impact the type of care you will receive. Immigrants from South Asian cultures, when settled into the West, are less likely to reach out for help because they are not able to resonate with the resources and support that is available to them in their new environment (Reichert, 2018). Due to this, immigrant families report high levels of stress and poor mental health, which can be detrimental as prolonged mental health struggles can develop into severe mental illnesses. This is where e-mental health can play a significant role in improving the lives of immigrants, or any individual, who wishes to access mental health services of a different culture or geographical region. E-mental health resources offer educational tools in various native languages making it easy to access information in non-native regions. One of the biggest concerns in the mental health care system is the access to quality and equitable care (Moock, 2014). E-mental health resources that are able to provide translations, connect people to resources in their homeland, and offer alternatives that closely resemble their culture, all bring a community closer to closing the gap and pitfalls that exist in delivering equitable and accessible care. Lastly, e-mental health resources also allow for continued patient care beyond the initial treatment phase (Moock, 2014). For example, the availability of various apps will help remind patients about their upcoming appointments or allow them to track their behaviours which is especially effective for those who are struggling with addiction and other behavioural disorders. The mental health apps serve as a connection between the patient and the clinician or therapist even after they have completed their in-person sessions. This sort of tracking and checking in resources help ensure the continued delivery of quality health care while serving as a tool that will help researchers monitor the efficacy of the treatment provided and how they can improve further interventions. The educational resources also provide virtual training and mental health certification programs that will enable citizens to learn how to identify someone who is struggling with their mental health and connect them to the help they need. It is not realistic to expect each individual in a community to attend in-person training and get certified as a general peer supporter. However, when these certifications are offered virtually, one can expect to have a large group of people take advantage of the accessibility of such programs and revolutionize the mental health landscape in their communities (Moock, 2014).

It is important to acknowledge the role e-mental health plays during the current COVID-19 pandemic (Situmorang, 2020). The COVID-19 pandemic has impacted human lives in drastic ways including how they communicate and connect with other people due to social isolation. Countries around the world have been placed under a lockdown with regulations enforcing people to work from home, study virtually and stay indoors (Situmorang, 2020). These restrictions alone have had adverse effects on the mental health of people as we are social human beings and the lack of social connection has resulted in depression, anxiety and stress related symptoms. Moreover, individuals who were already diagnosed with mental illness and those who were struggling with their mental health before the pandemic are now facing much severe circumstances as their treatment settings and overall coping environment has been drastically impacted by the coronavirus (Situmorang, 2020). Unfortunately, with the government issued restrictions in place, mental health services are no longer delivered face to face/in-person as counselors, psychologists, spiritual healers and pastorals were all requested to maintain physical distancing measures which prevented them from continuing their services via the normal in-person method. All around the world, psychiatrists, counselors, spiritual healers and peer supporters adapted to cyber counselling which is a form of online counseling done via texting services, video call or voice call. Such form of online counselling has proven to be the best solution amidst the COVID-19 pandemic and this highlights another great strength of e-mental health in the context of the current global pandemic. The rise in mental health related issues due to the pandemic also resulted in a rise in the number of people who are accessing helplines. One important aspect of e-mental health that has come to attention is that perhaps the option of staying anonymous while reaching out for help and being in one's own comfort zone might be linked to better mental health outcomes and thus such e-mental health resources might be beneficial in the post-pandemic world as well (Situmorang, 2020).

With any service or resource, oftentimes despite the numerous benefits, there may be contraindications that can raise some concerns and doubts about the service or resource (Wise et al, 2018). This is also the case for e-mental health. While we have discussed various different strengths and benefits of e-mental health, such as treatment and early interventions options, access to equitable healthcare, educational tools and the COVID-19 friendly services, there also exists some potential threats and drawbacks that are just as important to discuss.

One of the main expectations patients have when accessing any sort of medical care is privacy and confidentiality (Wise et al, 2018). Maintaining confidentiality and privacy is the right of every patient and the responsibility of the physician. These regulations are in effect when accessing mental health resources as well. Surprisingly, the expectations of patients for the protection of their privacy and confidence is much stronger when accessing mental health services perhaps due to the stigma associated with mental illness and psychological treatments. However, e-mental health relies on various different virtual platforms that are designed by different software companies and are not necessarily established by the healthcare provider themselves (Wise et al, 2018). Due to the involvement of third party platforms in the process of delivering care, it is crucial that people are aware about the potential pitfalls and gaps that may exist in the system and it is important to perform thorough analysis on exactly how patient confidentiality and privacy is maintained on these virtual operating platforms (Wise et al, 2018).

Another follow up concern to privacy and confidentiality is the process of record keeping (Wise et al, 2018). In any healthcare area, including mental health and mental illness, patient records play an important role in ensuring that patient information is up-to-date as it helps with future diagnosis, transferring or referring patients to other mental health facilities and clinicians, and for the patient themselves. However, when these records are saved online, there is a higher risk of them being transferred to other users or destroyed since they are saved as soft copied instead of hard copies. The possibility of patient records being transferred online is very risky since it can pose a threat to patient confidentiality and privacy as mentioned earlier (Wise et al, 2018). As more users are turning towards e-mental health resources and services due to our current circumstances, it is crucial that the government and policy makers enforce a new law that places an increased emphasis on the protection of patient records especially ones that are being saved electronically (Wise et al, 2018). Lastly, it is important to understand that in psychological treatments and interventions such as therapy and peer support groups, human connection plays a crucial role in the process of healing and recovery (Moock, 2014). E-mental health services, while accessible to a larger group of people, do lack the human connection which was established by being in the same physical space (Moock, 2014).

Therefore, it is important to physicians, clinicians, counselors, therapists, spiritual healers and other mental health professionals to constantly take in feedback from their patients when delivering services electronically in order to ensure that the standards of care are not being compromised (Moock, 2014).

In conclusion, e-mental health resources and services are a great tool for revolutionizing the mental health landscape in communities. They provide a virtual platform for treatments and interventions that help patients receive diagnosis and treatment in a timely manner while also providing educational resources that are an asset in raising mental health awareness and educating people about mental health literacy. Moreover, e-mental health has played a crucial role in the light of the COVID-19 pandemic as it has been the service that millions of people around the world have turned towards for the betterment of their mental health. While the benefits are very promising, it is important to reflect on the possible contraindications on e-mental health and how any sort of gaps and pitfalls in the electronic system can pose a threat to confidentiality and privacy of the patient. However, these gaps can be addressed with proper considerations. It is also important to note that accessing mental health services and resources in the form of e-mental health may be fairly recent for many individuals and so it is important that people are comfortable and are able to connect despite the lack of human connection compared to in-person services.

Overall, the benefits definitely outweigh the risks that were discussed in this chapter and hence e-mental health has a lot of potential of filling in the gaps that exist in our current mental health care system.

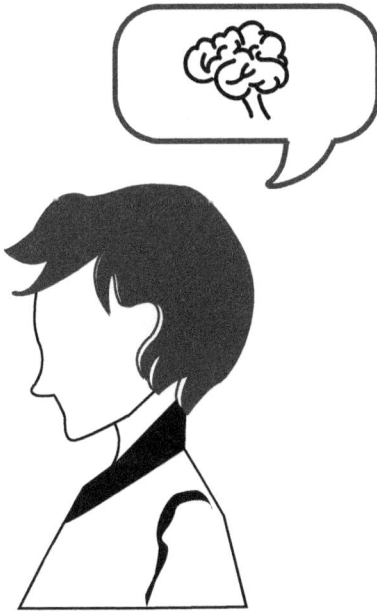

The Science of E-mental Health

Angelina Lam

An Introduction to the Science of Mental Health

E-mental health, as introduced in earlier chapters, encompasses the wide-spanning idea of using the internet and online technologies in relation to the field of mental health (Riper et al., 2010). Science is a fundamental aspect of mental health research; thus, science also plays an important part in e-mental health interventions and initiatives. This is because scientific literature forms the basis of how mental health professionals approach and develop practices. Although an online setting may reimagine the method of delivery, e-mental health still draws from research in a multitude of scientific fields such as psychology, neuroscience, biology, mathematics, and computer science. This new paradigm of online mental healthcare exemplifies the need to better integrate and understand multiple scientific disciplines.

To preface the importance of science in e-mental health, first, science in traditional mental health must be explored. Psychology, first and foremost, plays a large role in mental health interventions. Psychology studies many ideas such as behaviour, cognition, perception, relationships, and more

(Wittchen et al., 2015). Psychological principles inform the human understanding of mental health and how to support it. From this, it also describes current knowledge on mental disorders and how to treat them with interventions (Wittchen et al., 2015). Evidence-based psychological interventions are utilized to treat a variety of disorders including mood disorders, anxiety disorders, and more (The Australian Psychological Society, 2018). It plays an important role due to its effectiveness in this capacity; however additional research can be conducted to further understand psychotherapy and how it is effective (Richardson, 1997; Wittchen et al., 2015).

Other fields of science also play an important role in the current research in mental health. For example, combinations of biology and neuroscience can also describe mental health processes. Cognitive neuroscience examines brain activity and juxtapositions it with cognitive processes to understand how they are interconnected (Pereira, 2007). It examines biomarkers and neural targets to tailor mental healthcare to individuals, relating brain changes to treatment responses (Wojtalik et al., 2018). For example, researchers have attempted to pinpoint specific signatures of the brain that may indicate a higher risk for mental health problems, or certain brain identifiers that would correlate to a better response to treatment. These discoveries help to pivot certain treatments to more efficient usages and overall contribute to growing research in mental healthcare (Cacioppo et al., 2007; Wojtalik et al.,

2018). Social neuroscience is also an emerging field that involves mental health (Cacioppo et al., 2007). Research in this field relates studies of the brain to social behaviour and mental health. A neuroscience-based understanding of social activity can inform researchers about the development of mental illnesses; however, this field is extremely interdisciplinary and promising progress will hopefully help overcome any challenges faced in research (Cacioppo et al., 2007).

A more focused concept in biology, the concept of genetics, has also been explored in relation to mental health. Familial genetics results in a connected risk of mental health issues (Hyman, 2000). This is due to how genetic information relates to cells, brain structures, proteins, and more, which may dictate the brain's response to drugs and disease. Some combinations of genetic variations may affect behaviour and increase or decrease the risks of mental disorders (Hyman, 2000). This idea is complicated and has many facets; genetic influences are not clear-cut and straightforward. Genetic factors interact between themselves as well as with environmental input. Their expression, as known as a phenotype, is difficult to characterize. Focuses on large genetic databases can allow for the studying of disease prevalences and illness prevention (Hyman, 2000).

On a population level, mental health also deals with the sciences of public health and overall population wellness. Mental health is directly tied to overall health, as the definition of health as described by the World Health Organization includes a full state of wellbeing in mental, physical, and social aspects (World Health Organization, 1948). Some research in this field includes psychiatric epidemiology, which uses epidemiological principles to study mental health in the wider population (Patten, 2015). Mental health can take on aspects of public health as well; examples include strategies to promote population wellness, the development of programs and policies, etc (Canadian Public Health Association, 2021). This illustrates the wide-encompassing range of sciences that mental health is connected with.

An Introduction to the Science of E-Mental Health

In terms of e-mental health, its fundamentals still require a multidisciplinary foundation in science. However, some aspects may be increased or decreased depending on the intervention's method of delivery. Shifting to an online format brings increased access to many populations despite geographical location or other barriers; it integrates information and communication technology (ICT) as an attempt to enhance care (Lal & Adair, 2014; Shoemaker & Hilty, 2016). There are many different types of delivery and adapted interventions. Crucial communication platforms in e-mental health include website-, videoconferencing-, and email-based interventions, while alternative platforms such as virtual reality and chats are also being used (OHTN Rapid Response Service, 2018). Despite its different methods of dissemination, much of the equivalent programming is still able to be implemented and thus, would be rooted in the sciences (Daigle & Rudnick, 2020).

The Psychological Background of E-Mental Health

To explore e-mental health, it is seen that both the intervention strategy as well as the method of delivery have implications in science. This section will explore a few select interventions and methods of ICT delivery. One popular method used online is cognitive behavioural therapy, also known as CBT. CBT is a method of psychotherapy that primarily focuses on helping the person question their beliefs, which leads to helping them change their outlook to a more positive one (Rector, 2010). By teaching a person to pinpoint misrepresentations of certain situations and to view them from a different point of view instead, this can change the way they approach the situation. If CBT is successful, the psychotherapy can help to alleviate problematic trains of thought (Rector, 2010).

Scientifically, CBT's understanding in psychology relates to a cognitive model in which people's perceptions are determinant of their emotion and behaviour (Fenn & Byrne, 2013). This is based on a model of human cognition, where it is outlined as: interactions between someone's core beliefs about people and the world, dysfunctional assumptions that they live by, and negative automatic thoughts (Fenn & Byrne, 2013). Using this three-level model, this defines an individual's experiences and problems, and allows the individual to be understood. As previously mentioned, this lets the therapist aid the patient in understanding their negative thoughts, which allows them to revise and overcome them. Some specific techniques include guided discovery to reach different conclusions about a scenario, recording thoughts to be aware of thoughts and emotions, etc (Fenn & Byrne, 2013). CBT helps treat disorders such as anxiety, post traumatic stress disorder, bipolar disorder, and more (Fenn & Byrne, 2013).

In terms of e-mental health, a number of reviews as well as studies have been conducted on internet cognitive behavioural therapy (iCBT). Instead of long wait times to access one-on-one CBT treatment, iCBT can offer a combination of self-initiated or therapist-led treatment while avoiding barriers to care (Lal, 2019). Studies have indicated that iCBT's success is akin to that of in-person CBT; they also mostly state that iCBT improves the mental health of those affected with anxiety and depression (Lal, 2019; OHTN Rapid Response Service, 2018). However, some studies have also found no significant changes in symptoms in cases of anxiety, depression, and suicide prevention (OHTN Rapid Response Service, 2018). Limited research restricts the ability to compare both iCBT and in-person CBT (Lal, 2019). This issue is prevalent in e-mental health as it is difficult to gather information on demographics as well as garner substantial follow-ups. It is also difficult to examine iCBT in different contexts of care; in primary care, a study found it to be effective, but more research is needed in these departments (Lal, 2019; Williams & Andrews, 2013). A case study of iCBT usage is shown by the MindSpot

Clinic, an Australian national e-mental health initiative visited by almost 500,000 people (Titov et al., 2017). Specifically, MindSpot enrolled people in one of their courses depending on their circumstances and mental health needs. Over eight weeks, those enrolled were presented with slides and principles on CBT, and at the end, outcomes were measured using several psychological scales, including those from the Diagnostic and Statistical Manual of Mental Disorders, 4th Edition (DSM IV) (Titov et al., 2017). Of the 70.5% of patients who had finished their treatment, 66.1% had completed the survey to measure outcomes. Out of MindSpot's four courses, symptom reductions for three were around 43.0% at the end of treatment and 52.3% after a three-month follow-up. For the last course, symptom reduction was found to be 25.5% post-treatment, rising to 27.5% after three months (Titov et al., 2017). This study showed that MindSpot was able to provide evidence-based treatment in regards to mental health even in an online environment (Titov et al., 2017). Satisfaction rates were high as well as patient engagement. It was able to reach a wide audience since 82% of users were not previously attaining mental health help and 35% have not contacted a mental health professional; the online treatment provided anonymity and easier access for those who had barriers to treatment (Titov et al., 2017). Though it fares well against in-person treatment, this case of iCBT delivery was not meant to replace it (Titov et al., 2017). However, MindSpot still shows the potential positive and time-saving impacts of e-mental health initiatives on the population.

It shows the ability to use traditional scientific and psychological principles in an online format.

Additional studies of web-based CBT have also been previously conducted. MoodGYM, another Australian platform, provided varied outcomes (OHTN Rapid Response Service, 2018). Reviews state that it had a high chance of having an impact but additional study into the topic was needed (OHTN Rapid Response Service, 2018). The University of Regina had also formed the Online Therapy Unit for Service Education and Research, which used iCBT to treat mental disorders such as anxiety and depression (Mental Health Commission of Canada, 2014). Their study had concluded iCBT helped their users' symptoms and that overall, the program increased reach and access to care in the province (Mental Health Commission of Canada, 2014). This depicts the popularity of iCBT platforms and some of the different research conducted to explore this topic.

However, websites and interactive experiences were not the only means of delivering CBT. Video conferencing, where counselling was performed through digital means, also commonly employed CBT strategies (OHTN Rapid Response Service, 2018). For many age groups, settings, and disorders, online counselling showed no significant differences to in-person therapy sessions (OHTN Rapid Response Service, 2018). Technological issues such as difficulty hearing or poor sound quality may negatively impact the experience; however, video conferencing is mostly met with highly satisfied participants (McGinty et al., 2006). Thus, it acts as another online format for mental health assistance.

Another psychology-related intervention is the idea of teaching patients and their family about the mental illness and treatments (Ekhtiari et al., 2017). This is done in an emotionally-cognisant and motivational way (Ekhtiari et al., 2017). This intervention, coined psychoeducation, equips patients with the knowledge to understand their illness, cope with it, feel motivated, and ultimately be more likely to follow through with treatment (Bäuml et al., 2006). Analysis of research identified that even brief passive psychoeducation can grant a positive outcome and reduce symptoms for conditions such as depression (Bäuml et al., 2006; Donker et al., 2009).

In e-mental health applications, psychoeducation can be provided by websites (Barak & Grohol, 2011). Various styles of disseminating this information include informational websites or tutorials. This type of therapy overall is effective and provides positive outcomes; it makes bibliotherapy, the use of literature to aid with mental illness, more accessible and available than ever (Barak & Grohol, 2011; Abdullah, 2005). Despite that, it is important to look for credible information, as some sources of mental health information were found to be misleading and lack citations (Barak & Grohol, 2011). Thus, psychoeducation through ICT platforms may bring positive impacts, but readers must stay vigilant on what sources are being used.

As for other avenues of mental health assistance, chat and email were also used. Synchronous text-based communication showed both positive and variable outcomes (OHTN Rapid Response Service, 2018). Email, on the other hand, is one of the most popular methods to provide online, individual therapy. Conclusions range from effective to mixed, but overall, it provides a convenient and asynchronous method of communication (Barak & Grohol, 2011; OHTN Rapid Response Service, 2018). It can be noted that email counselling can act as a gateway to face-to-face counselling, as an email format may be more casual and less stigmatizing (Schmidt & Wykes, 2012). However, for both methods, nonverbal cues are missing from both parties involved. Psychologically, nonverbal cues such as posture and facial expression play an important role in communicating feelings in a social interaction (Riggio & Riggio, 2012). Thus, email or text-based therapy has advantages and disadvantages that must be considered (Barak & Grohol, 2011).

Additional Scientific Aspects of E-Mental Health

As interdisciplinary as mental health is, e-mental health is not an exception as it encompasses skills and tools from a variety of disciplines. To briefly touch upon some fields, mathematics, computer science, and public health all play a role in this electronic counterpart. Some have become more prevalent than others due to a change in scope of information and practices.

Mathematics, to start, already plays a crucial role

in statistical analyses even during in-person mental health studies. In e-mental health, this role may include large data sets of online users. As an example, the aforementioned MindSpot Clinic had regularly amassed website data, with 500,000 visits and 25,469 sets of data for analysis (Titov et al., 2017). Statistical analysis was crucial to determine if there were significant therapeutic outcomes or effects. Data science can also be used to survey certain populations on mental health opinions and demographic information, which can help professionals determine how to best serve a population (Lal, 2019). In addition, sets of data from a person's activity can be used to assess risks for suicide or homicide (Mental Health Commission of Canada, 2014). With the advent of social media, this also provides a range of data capable of being analyzed in the e-mental health realm. There are, however, ethical considerations needed in cases such as these (Mental Health Commission of Canada, 2014).

Moreover, some of this data collection is made possible by advances in technology and computer science. Without revolutionary strides in the development of technology, e-mental health would not exist. With that technology comes a greater ability to monitor and assess mental health outcomes (Bauer & Moessner, 2012). This can be used to provide more personalized feedback due to an increased frequency of assessments and computer-analyzed answers (Schmidt & Wykes, 2012). Additionally, usability and design of software are enormous factors that are dictated by computer science and engineering (Becker, 2016).

This introduces a crucial aspect of care that can help increase adherence rates and outcomes (Becker, 2016).

Furthermore, computer science can pioneer novel tools to aid with psychological analyses. Machine learning, for example, involves both mathematics and computer science to assist professionals in finding patterns in clinical data (Becker, 2016). By analyzing survey and outcome data, among other data sets, computer science can help increase the efficiency of e-mental health. This is because machine learning can be used to predict outcomes, diagnose disorders, or recommend therapies. Technology is improving and further research can show that this may be applied to different methods of care, whether it be facial emotion or text-based analyses (Becker, 2016).

New platforms are also being explored in relation to e-mental health. Mobile technology can help to identify activities of a patient, where a lull in activity may be an indication to check the patient for signs of depression (Becker, 2016). Wearable technologies can track physiological data such as sleep habits, pulses, mood, and location, which can grant professionals data for analysis and treatment plans (Mental Health Commission of Canada, 2014). Virtual reality and video games are also novel means of providing interactive mental healthcare. For example virtual reality can simulate ideas or conditions that would aid someone in overcoming anxiety or post traumatic stress disorder (Mental Health Commission of Canada, 2014). Video games may employ the same principle to replicate an environment for clients to deal with certain issues; for example, the game Playmancer was developed to help players deal with problematic impulse issues when related to gambling (Schmidt & Wykes, 2012). This shows the relevance of computer science in the future of e-mental health.

In a public health and population studies context, e-mental health seems to generally encourage a more widespread and accessible gateway to mental health support (Lal, 2019). This is because rural populations can increasingly access these services despite the distance barrier (Mental Health Commission of Canada, 2014). Youth are also a demographic that may benefit from digitized mental health initiatives since an Irish study stated that 68% would be willing to use internet-based mental health support (Mental Health Commission of Canada, 2014). However, it must be kept in mind that those without internet access will be left behind; it is important to consider the social determinants of healthcare and how to best design a system that will still address the needs of those who do not have internet access or are not able to access the web due to severe mental illnesses (Mental Health Commission of Canada, 2014). Thus, e-mental health encompasses population sciences in considering its delivery.

Conclusion

In conclusion, e-mental health is a wholly multidisciplinary topic spanning many of the sciences, including psychology, neuroscience, biology, mathematics, computer science, and public health. Through exploring many scientific aspects of its implementation, from converting interventions to digital formats, to developing feasible software solutions, to ensuring accurate and fair access, there are many questions that arise regarding how to best implement an integrated online system (Titov et al., 2017). E-mental health is promising and introduces many considerations that need to be addressed with an online care model. However, considerable progress has been made as its delivery continues to improve. Thus, further research in this field through multiple scientific disciplines will aid this process. The resultant trials will ultimately lead the action on how to best continue implementing e-mental healthcare worldwide.

The Reliability and Skepticism Around E-mental Health

Maria Ashraf

As previous chapters explored the significance and background of e-mental health, the subsequent step in understanding its potential application is examining its reliability. Reliability for e-mental health can be assessed and viewed in several ways. It can look like anything from using accurate resources for curating a mental health website to designing rigorous clinical trials to assess telepsychiatry interventions. However, in essence, these services should be able to accurately and reliably accomplish their said objectives while being safe for clients to utilize. In terms of reliability, there is considerable empirical evidence that many e-mental health services are safe and reliable (Mucic & Hilty, 2016). However, despite the current evidence for the advocacy of e-mental health, there exists some secondary factors that impact its reliability and safety. Issues such as scope of practice, regulation, risk management, etc. are important to discuss. Additionally, this chapter will also define reliability through its role in the development and delivery of e-mental health, and its comparative efficacy to traditional approaches.

To begin, properly assessing the reliability of e-mental health can prove to be a complex task when considering the relatively recent spike in technological advancements and e-mental health services. While technology has given rise to innovative opportunities for e-mental health, the development of research and regulations has not kept up at the same pace. This has consequently resulted in an unfortunate lack of unanimous regulatory organizations that can provide unified regulation of e-mental health (E-Mental Health in Canada, 2014). However, this does not imply an absolute lack of regulation of e-mental health services either. There are present various established and emerging approaches to regulate e-mental health services. For example, in Canada, national and provincial psychological organizations have come up with appropriate standards and specific models for regulation of e-mental health services such as telepsychology and teletherapy (Association of Canadian Psychology Regulatory Organizations (ACPRO), 2011). Additionally, with a surge in mobile based e-mental health, there is ongoing research in designing necessary frameworks to accurately assess different mental health apps. One example is a framework that was developed by Canadian psychologists that mapped out nine principles to assess the reliability of mental health apps to help guide healthcare professionals in their decisions (Zelmer et al., 2018). In essence, most of the work and established guidelines about the reliability of e-mental health services typically comes from literature and empirical studies. However, when it comes to assigning the ultimate responsibility of objectively assessing reliability, it is challenging to designate it to a unified source. Oftentimes, navigating the reliability of specific e-mental health services can inevitably become the responsibility of the caregiver or patient themselves.

Additionally, when assessing the reliability of e-mental health services, it is important to realize the specific limitations of e-mental health services and the intended scope of their application. E-mental health services have varied intended uses and are not recommended for all aspects of mental health or for all groups of people. This limited use also has implications for safety and scope of practice. For example, online therapy platforms like Talkspace are able to provide therapy sessions for a variety of mental health issues (Talkspace, 2021). However, such platforms are unable to provide teletherapy to younger age groups i.e. younger than 13 years. Thus, making them non-functional for children. On the other hand, websites like e-mentalhealth.ca only aim to inform patients about different mental health resources. These platforms are not capable of treating mental health conditions (eMentalHealth.ca, 2021). This indicates that not all e-mental health services are well equipped or compatible with all types of mental health concerns. Consequently, e-mental health may not represent a safe or reliable option for every mental health concern either. This highlights that while e-mental health is a promising option in expanding mental health service, it is not an alternative or replacement to traditional services (E-Mental Health in Canada, 2014). Therefore, before exploring the reliability and safety of any e-mental health service, it is necessary to adequately explore its appropriateness and intended use.

With those considerations in mind, let's briefly explore the development and systematics underlying e-mental health services and their impact on reliability. As discussed in the previous chapter, the systems and principles underlying most e-mental health services are rooted in scientific literature and are additionally based upon psychological guidelines. This is especially true for services that engage in therapeutic and clinical practices. For example, in order to design an e-mental health service, there is emphasis on utilizing evidence based models and systems. The Canadian Mental Health Commission recently carried out its annual summary report and emphasized the need for incorporating evidence-based practices for e-mental health services (Mental Health Commission of Canada, 2020). Likewise, in terms of research, there are several journals, articles, and studies dedicated to internet based therapy and health. The journal of medical internet research being a notable example, which includes various studies on e-mental health (JIMR, 2021). Another aspect of e-mental health reliability is the utilization of user experience in the development of services. The added benefit of harnessing contemporary technology can be accompanied with the downside of reduced usability and effectiveness. Hence, it is essential that e-mental health services are assessed for the variable of user experience. This emphasis has been taken into account in various e-mental health studies and interventions. For instance, the digital program SMART, that deals with mild traumatic brain injury was updated and redesigned according to user inputs in terms of its usability and experience. Overall, this led to increased reliability and efficacy of the service (Schmidt et al., 2020). Similarly, a study done on improving internet-based Cognitive Behavioural Therapy (CBT) focused on a user-centered evaluation approach to understand how patients assessed the service (Geirhos et al., 2021). This was also done to improve the reliability of the intervention. Therefore, the themes of incorporating empirical data and creating opportunities in the research and development of e-mental health are heavily promoted and emphasized by e-mental health researchers and providers. This reliance and utilization of evidence based systems serve as a primer and framework towards developing reliable e-mental health services.

Furthermore, a crucial aspect that attests to the reliability of e-mental health is the systems in place for its administration to clients. As discussed earlier, there are several methodologies and applications of e-mental health. Some services may be self-regulated while others rely on supervision and collaboration between therapists and clients. Services that incorporate blended approaches are highly dependent on evidence based models (Mental Health Commission of Canada, 2020). Additionally, the services are provided by trained and licensed mental healthcare providers. For example, one of the most researched and applied forms of e-mental health is i-CBT (Internet-Delivered Cognitive

Behavioural Therapy). A study examining iCBT administration across 5 European and North American countries highlighted several measures in place to assure patient safety and treatment. Specifically, the study explores a iCBT clinic in Canada that has set guidelines, frameworks, and registered mental health providers or other related trained professionals to deliver treatment. Additionally, each treatment had policies and regulations that were in accordance with the nation's standard healthcare practices. This need for standardization and regulation advances into the information and educational e-mental health services. As discussed earlier in this chapter there are current and upcoming regulatory bodies to assess specific e-mental health services. However, within some of the current services there has been an increase in validating sources and using evidence based approaches. For example, the Canadian Centre for Addiction and Mental Health only recommends a select few mental health mobile applications and applies a rigorous selecting mechanism. Specifically, it looks at the presence of evidence and privacy protocols (CAMH, 2021). Similarly, the American Psychology Association, has come up with an app advisor model to improve physicians selection of e-mental health apps. It also emphasizes clinical foundations and safety as some of its key evaluators (APA, 2021). Similarly, there have also been studies that review the effectiveness of mental health services such as informational websites like ementalhealth.ca (Jeong et al., 2019). Overall, the reliability and safety of delivery systems in place for the majority of e-mental health services are for the most part, assessed through empirical data and research.

After exploring the systematical and administrative reliability of e-mental health, this chapter will move on to understand reliability in terms of efficacy. In order to assess the reliability of e-mental health, it is important to compare it to the efficacy of traditional care. Traditional mental healthcare embodies rigorous trial and testing through clinical trials, overall engaging in an evidence-based approach. This same approach has been implemented to appraise the reliability of e-mental health services through literature reviews and empirical studies. The current literature on e-mental health efficacy can be broadly categorized into 1) testing specific interventions and 2) evaluating educational resources and other supplementary services. Beginning with the literature on the efficacy of e-mental health interventions, there is substantial evidence in favour of e-mental health. Several reviews and trials have concluded that these interventions produce similar results to traditional care. A review done on 75 papers on telemental health found it to be beneficial in addressing a variety of mental health issues such as depression, schizophrenia, post traumatic stress disorders (PTSD), eating disorders, and panic disorders (Hailey et al., 2008). Furthermore, one of the areas of mental health that have greatly utilized several e-mental health services is depression and anxiety concerns. There is a substantial amount of evidence that maintains the efficacy of e-mental health services such as iCBT and other forms of teletherapy for depression and anxiety issues. Several studies mention that it was as effective as face-to-face interaction in achieving clinical outcomes (Andersson & Hedman, 2013; Ruwaard et al., 2012; Stjerneklar et al., 2019). The evidence in favour of e-mental health also extends to other mental health concerns. Several clinical trials have highlighted the efficacy of e-mental health in treating patients with PTSD (Gaebel, 2017). There is also growing evidence for treatment of panic disorders and eating disorders (Schlegl et al., 2015). Additionally, another area of testing the efficacy of e-mental health services is testing the reliability of assessment and administration methods. Several studies done on psychological testing through virtual means have highlighted their reliability in assessing patients as effectively as in-person assessments (Chakrabarti, 2015; Hubely et al., 2016). Additionally, there is also evidence on the reliability of techniques such as videoconferencing. A critical review done on video conferencing in e-mental health found it to be reliable and efficient (Chakrabarti, 2015). Furthermore, the efficacy of e-mental health services extends to the information based services as well. There is also evidence that highlights the benefits of information based systems such as e-mental health applications and websites (Chandrashekar, 2018). Similarly, there is growing evidence in favour of e-mental health services like systems based on artificial intelligence systems that help improve detection and therapeutic systems (Ćosić et al., 2020 ; D'Alfonso, 2020).

Even with considerable evidence in favour of e-mental health services, skepticism and concerns regarding the reliability of e-mental health do exist. While these beliefs are not indubitable rejections of e-mental health services, they can be categorized as a series of concerns regarding the application and reliability of e-mental health. Additionally, these beliefs may originate from a variety of different sources. Caregivers may have concerns regarding the specifics of treatment and nature of e-mental health. Similarly, clients may not be comfortable or feel safe while using e-mental health. Lastly, there might be opposition from research bodies that may have issues with the fairly recent nature of e-mental health.

Firstly, a major concern in terms of the reliability of e-mental health is the nature of virtual platforms and concerns with privacy. Healthcare providers might find it difficult to provide reliable and safe treatment in unique virtual settings. This is especially relevant for services where the client remains anonymous. While this anonymity has been seen to be beneficial for the client, it can be concerning for caregivers. The lack of transparency leaves room for the inability of caregivers to authenticate that they are communicating with their client (Harris & Birnbaum, 2015). This can have implications of not being able to assess whether a client's progress is their own or to form a relationship with the client. In addition, client's may find virtual platforms and their privacy policies to be concerning in terms of how their data is used. Some components of e-mental health branch out of the patient-provider settings and incorporate external forces into their systems. This can include partnerships with firms involved in the design and conveyance of virtual services such as Artificial Intelligence, business, software designing etc. The incorporation of third parties can raise concerns about data security and the overall safety of these systems (Stoll, et al., 2020).

An additional concern regarding the reliability of e-mental health mainly stems from reduced or complete omission of face-to-face interaction. This is a concern highlighted mainly by caregivers that find face-to face interaction essential in building a therapeutic alliance with their clients. A therapeutic alliance is considered an integral part of therapeutic interventions (Tremain et al., 2020). In a study done on the perceptions of caregivers for video conferencing, it was concluded that they felt that they could not adequately form a therapeutic alliance with their client which has impacts on the overall effectiveness of the therapy (Chakrabarti, 2015; Wade et al., 2015). Additionally, they indicated a need for real time processing of a clients non-verbal cues that they require for providing adequate therapy. Furthermore, due to their personal preferences and expertise, many healthcare professionals are reluctant to reestablish their practices to incorporate e-health (Mayer et al., 2019). This lack of direct and immediate connection also acts as a concern that e-mental health is not safe to be used for mental health concerns that require vigilant risk management. Many caregivers have pointed out the lack of concrete risk management strategies to be a major reason for their relecuntancy to adopt e-mental health services. Similarly, risk management cannot be carried out attentively and promptly in certain e-mental health services which make them an unsafe option for certain mental health issues (Andersson & Titov, 2014). Specifically, e-mental health is not advised for patients dealing with psychosis or suicide ideation.

An additional factor to be considered in assessing the reliability of e-mental health services lies in the use of the internet. There is no doubt that the recent development and enhancement of e-mental health services could not be done without the aid and contribution of the internet. The internet has led to an increased use and awareness of e-mental health. However, this same wide spread use can become a problem in terms of reliability. This is especially relevant to e-mental health services that are unregulated and clients access them unsupervised. This can include social media, peer-to-peer forums, blogs, and informative websites. Since there is a lack of regulatory services, these sources of e-mental health can be prone to being inaccurate. Not only does this have implications for inaccuracy, the nature of these sources can lead to misinformation and issues such as anxiety due to self diagnosis. The lack of regulation in these services can greatly reduce their reliability and make platforms that can undermine safety and accuracy.

Lastly, an additional concern highlighted by critics of the reliability of e-mental health is the paucity of available research. While there is an abundance and continued growth of evidence in favour of e-mental health, there are also some issues within the use of these services. For example, for some e-mental health intervention studies the attrition rates can be high. Many patients enrolled in clinical trials dropout before the completion of the intervention. Some studies have tried to explore the connection between attrition rates and efficacy of treatments. They look at what are some characteristics of patients that help them remain in trials and continue treatment. They also look at whether any economic or literacy factors come into play (Al-Asadi et al., 2016). This can lead to concerns on how these rates impact the reliability of the results. It highlights the issue that maybe these interventions are only effective for a certain group of patients. This lack of evidence can sometimes also lead to hesitancy in mental healthcare providers before fully adopting e-mental health.

Overall, e-mental health services are an important step forward in improving the accessibility and features of mental health services. A considerable part of these advancements can be attributed to the novel and exponential growth of the technological and virtual communications sectors. As innovative and constructive this is, this rapid pace of advancement has also led to concerns regarding the reliability and safety of e-mental health services. To tackle the issue of reliability, there is considerable existing and growing evidence supporting the efficacy of e-mental health services. Additionally, there is also a shift in setting up regulations and standards to assess the reliability of e-mental health. Despite this, there still are concerns regarding the efficacy and reliability of e-mental health. These concerns can tie back to the decisions and understandings of caregivers and patients. However, there is hope that with growing evidence and regulatory bodies, the overall skepticism and concerns can be reduced. In essence, e-mental health services are sustained by a great deal of evidence in practice and literature making it a reliable and safe option for various mental health concerns. Furthermore, building upon the theme of safety, the next chapter will further explore e-mental health and how it contributes to creating safe and accessible environments.

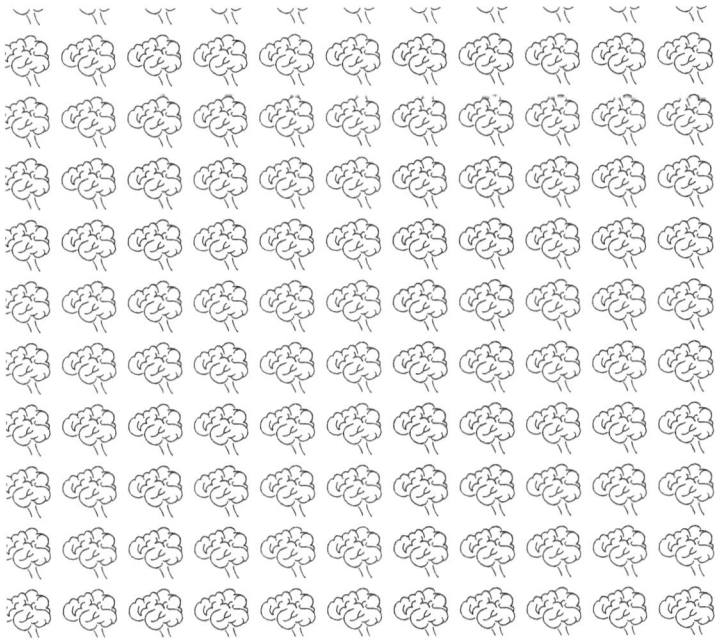

E-mental Health: A Safe Environment for Everyone

Madiha Ansari

Since there are many individuals who are in need of help regarding their mental health, e-mental health has become an effective and accessible resource for everyone. Therefore, e-mental health is organized in a way which allows a safe environment for every individual; it aspires to be a welcoming resource which makes one feel comfortable and safe when talking about their mental health. Furthermore, mental health is an issue which affects every type of person; no matter what their gender, age, culture, or religion is. Hence, e-mental health provides a safe environment where people can freely talk about their mental health. Due to the advancements in technology and an increase in the awareness for mental health, countries around the world have taken steps to improve and moderate the help that is provided online. For instance, in Canada, many organizations have developed apps that provide assistance. Some of these examples are Mindfulness Coach, PTSD Coach Canada, and WHO Academy (CAMH, 2018). These resources are among the many other applications that are available online. Additionally, these applications are designed to be safe and confidential for all individuals. PTSD

Coach Canada, for example, emphasizes the security of the individuals who are using the application (Veterans Affairs Canada, 2019). Similarly, most of the resources for e-mental health are provided with certain policies and conditions that allow an individual to feel secure and safe when they are seeking help.

Henceforth, people are beginning to prefer e-mental health resources over in-person help, due to the ease and anonymity it provides. The reason behind this preference is the stigma that revolves around mental health. Many individuals avoid getting help because of their own, or the society's, stigmatized views; it is not due to a lack of care (Clement et al., 2012). Furthermore, individuals tend to have self-stigma when dealing with mental health issues (Wallin et al., 2018). For instance, they develop a stereotypical mindset such as a fear of social exclusion and feeling of shame, which prevents them from seeking help (Luoma et al., 2008). In particular, males who belong to an ethnic minority group, and youth, are two different groups of people who avoid receiving professional help for mental health issues (Wallin et al., 2018). Therefore, electronic mental health (e-mental health) was introduced as a way to approach individuals with self-stigma towards seeking help for their mental health problems. The possibility of having anonymity over a face-to-face conversation can overcome people's avoidance towards mental health issues (Clement et al., 2015). The ease and safety provided by this method, where treatment can be accessible on phones and computers, highlights the privacy that is involved (Wallin et al.,

2018). For instance, an individual can get treated in the privacy and safety of their own house, instead of having to face an unfamiliar person or setting. Moreover, the study conducted by Wallin et al. (2015), investigating the "Self-stigma and the intention to seek psychological help online compared to face-to-face", provided results suggesting that individuals, who had self-stigma regarding mental health, were not in-avoidance of getting help (Wallin et al., 2018). The study also found that individuals with higher levels of self-stigma also had higher intentions to seek online treatment (Wallin et al., 2018). Thus, the safety, privacy, and anonymity behind e-mental health can be supported by these studies. Undoubtedly, individuals who are uncomfortable when facing a stranger, can find it difficult to talk to them about their issues. Which is why, when therapists are helping people online, they tend to follow the process of texting, so that people can get comfortable and less hesitant to talk to them about their mental health issues (Andersson & Titov, 2014).

In the past two years, there has been a drastic change in the way the world used to work. COVID-19 has impacted a lot of things and having accessible mental health help is one of them. Due to the lack of interaction between humans, and the fear of coronavirus, many organizations were forced to halt their in-person treatments. Consequently, many individuals who sought help for their mental health issue were also impacted by the sudden change and lack of in-person help available. Along with that, due to the pandemic, there was an elevation in the amount of psychological distress in many people (Ho CS et al., 2020). Since the majority of mental health care was provided in hospitals, the pandemic caused many facilities to close down (Al-Alawi et al., 2021). Hence, e-mental health became an effective and accessible resource for many people. Individuals who had a specific therapist, and were comfortable with them, are now able to talk to them online and continue getting their help. Due to an increase in the ethical issues regarding e-mental health, many practitioners prioritized having face-to-face treatment, despite e-mental health being available for many years (Berger T., 2017). Nonetheless, e-mental health services have shown to be much effective when it comes to anxiety and depression; many individuals obtain positive outcomes when going through the process of online therapy (Karyotaki E et al., 2018). Furthermore, due to the coronavirus and its impacts, there is an increase in the demand for e-mental health (Wind TR et al., 2020). Consequently, many individuals are unable to access e-mental health services due to issues such as economic problems or network connectivity problems (Al-Alawi et al., 2021). Henceforth, there is an increase in the online resources such as applications and websites, that provide many individuals with free mental health care support and remedies to handle the amount of psychological distress during the pandemic (Al-Alawi et al., 2021). Thus, the online resources are made available and safe for every individual.

Technological advancements in health care have given rise to many new products and innovations.

Wearable devices are one of the new technologies that have been introduced; they monitor the mental health of an individual. These devices allow the person to have an all-time access to monitor their mental health (Nicholas et al., 2017). The wearable devices include many different features which help an individual keep track of their mental state. For instance, the device has breathing sensors, body signal monitoring, and heart rate monitors (Hunkin et al., 2020). When using a wearable device, the individual is able to hear sounds that switch between being calm to being intense (Hunkin et al., 2020). These sounds depend on the breathing of the wearer. Henceforth, an individual is able to obtain attention without anyone being present around them to judge or monitor them (Balconi et al., 2017). Thus, the wearable device is effective since it provides more privacy and tracks progress all the time; an individual is able to feel safe within their own space (Balconi et al., 2017). To add on, the study conducted by Hunkin et al. (2020), which investigated "Perceived acceptability of wearable devices for the treatment of mental health problems", suggested that individuals preferred having a monitoring wearable device as much as having talk therapies alone (Hunkin et al., 2020). As mentioned before, this device which is one of the techniques for e-mental health help, allows an individual, who self-stigmatizes mental health, to obtain help for their mental health problem (Hunkin et al., 2020). Moreover, this study also found that many individuals preferred a wearable device over other treatment options due to factors such as privacy and personal space (Hunkin et al., 2020). Hence, e-mental health has many different ways in which people can seek treatment without having to face or talk to another person. Although it is encouraged for an individual to discuss their mental health problems with a therapist, e-mental health allows that individual to at least take the first step into seeking professional help. Therefore, the treatment provided through e-mental health is designed to be safe and inclusive for everyone.

The increase in the awareness of mental health around the world has made a lot of countries consider and improve their resources for e-mental health. The research conducted by Meurk et al. (2016) on "Establishing and Governing e-Mental Health Care in Australia: A Systematic Review of Challenges and A Call For Policy-Focussed Research", talks about the current and future directions for e-mental health policy development in Australia (Meurk et al., 2016). Currently, many mental health researchers believe that e-mental health care is an effective and accessible resource which can be used to reach people all around the world (Meurk et al., 2016). Due to the increase in demand, mental health researchers have approached the government to support the technology behind e-mental health (Batterham PJ et al., 2015). Furthermore, these researchers are taking steps to ensure viable e-mental health services and e-therapies (Batterham PJ et al., 2015). However, it is inevitable that the increase in e-mental health services would impact face-to-face treatments all around the world (Meurk et al., 2016). Nonetheless, the potential of e-mental health can help more individuals as compared to face-to-face therapy sessions. This is because new technologies are being introduced into the health care system (Meurk et al., 2016), whereas old technologies are being innovated. Since the aim of e-mental health is to create a safe and accessible environment for everyone, technologies need to be developed in a way which incorporates the preferences of the individuals using it (Meurk et al., 2016). For instance, an individual needs easement and comfort when they use a certain type of technology. They do not want to have other technological issues while they are dealing with their mental health problems. Therefore, many factors need to be considered in order to make e-mental health safe and easy for everyone as well as having the capability to interact with therapists ethically. Hence, in order to develop technologies for e-mental health, a lot of mechanisms, scopes, and limits need to be identified and implemented to make e-mental health as effective and helpful as possible (Meurk et al., 2016). Thus, researchers analysed every factor which may prevent e-mental health services from helping others. For example, psychological, environmental, knowledge, and sociodemographic issues were all accounted for when improving the e-mental health services (Meurk et al., 2016). Overall, the aim of the researchers was to ensure a safe, accessible, and helpful e-mental health platform for everyone. E-mental health has become very important in the past few years. Regardless of the numerous amount of resources present, the number of people who get treatment for mental health remains small. One of the big issues regarding mental health care is that despite the numerous amount of people who struggle with mental health issues, 35% to 75% of the people, in high-income countries, are unable to get any type of treatment (Saxena S et al., 2015). Whereas in low and middle income countries, 76% to 85% of the people, struggling with mental health issues, are unable to get treatment (Saxena S et al., 2015). As mentioned previously, there are many reasons as to why people do not get professional treatment. Some of the examples include self-stigma, confidentiality issues, negative experiences, and unawareness of the resources available (Salaheddin K et al., 2016). Therefore, e-mental health has become popular in four different areas online: "self-guided web-based interventions, standalone mental health mobile apps, online peer support groups or interventions, and web-based counseling with registered professionals" (Alvarez-Jimenez et al., 2020). Web-based interventions is one of the areas which provided more negative outcomes. For example, the design of these interventions were made in order to replace face-to-face interventions, however, it resulted in less effectiveness and little innovation in technology, which was used to help people (Mohr et al., 2017). Meanwhile, the usage of mobile applications, which are based on mental health, increased during the past few years (Alvarez-Jimenez et al., 2020). However, these mental health mobile applications have had small effects on people's mental health. This issue most probably occurs due to the poor adherence (Baumel A et al., 2019) and lack of attention to keep the application and its features updated (Weisel KK et al., 2019). It was found that most mobile applications, targeted towards mental health, have been designed without taking clinical services into account, hence, giving non-effective results (Mohr et al., 2017). Online peer support groups are one of the other examples of e-mental health. Specially for young people who have mental health issues, peer-to-peer contact, along with therapeutic support, have allowed them to build a strong preference for online peer support groups (Lederman R et al., 2014). Nonetheless, the majority of these support groups lack the professional and clinical support, as well as the web-based therapy (Alvarez-Jimenez et al., 2020). Web-based counseling is another type of e-mental health service which is the most effective. Web-based counseling allows therapeutic alliance and face-to-face therapy (Richards D et al., 2013). However, due to the vast amount of individuals who need support, and because web-based counseling is a one-on-one support system, there is a lack of space for a lot of people to get treatment. Therefore, by considering the flaws in all four types of systems, researchers, Alvarez-Jimenez et al. (2020), have developed an innovative model called "Moderated Online Social Therapy (MOST)" (Alvarez-Jimenez et al., 2020). This model is created from merging all four types of e-mental health services in one; having effective and successful results (Alvarez-Jimenez et al., 2020). Furthermore, the same researchers have also introduced a new model called "Enhanced Moderated Online Social Therapy (MOST+)", which is targeted towards the young generations and their preferences (Alvarez-Jimenez et al., 2020). The two models, MOST and MOST+, considered the effective factors behind the web-based interventions, mobile applications, online peer support groups, and web-based counseling, to create a single platform; making it accessible and safe for every individual (Alvarez-Jimenez et al., 2020).

In conclusion, e-mental health provides accessible, safe, and private help for individuals with mental health issues. Hence, people started to prefer e-mental health; whether it was due to the issues behind COVID-19 or self-stigma. Since e-mental health provides a certain type of anonymity, people are able to communicate openly as compared to facing an unfamiliar person. Furthermore, one of the most effective reasons behind e-mental health is that it provides a safe environment for everyone. There is no discrimination, prejudice, or stereotype against individuals with different ethnicities, age, religions, etc. Undoubtedly, most face-to-face mental health treatments include these policies and beliefs too. However, a face-to-face interaction may make an individual feel intimidated or hesitant due to the differences between them and their therapist. Therefore, e-mental health is more effective when it involves a person to communicate about their personal problems. These are the reasons why many countries around the world have contributed to make e-mental health better. Furthermore, the rising awareness behind mental health issues have given many individuals an opportunity to express and talk about their problems. Additionally, as the stigma and negative stereotypes behind mental health decreases, people who willingly seek help for their mental health issues have increased. The safe environment, which surrounds e-mental health, is progressively making people get treatment for their mental health problems instead of disregarding them. With rising e-mental health platforms online, many ethical issues have arisen as well. Therefore, in the next chapter, the ethical and legal issues that are involved with e-mental health would be discussed more in-depth.

Ethics, Confidentiality, and Legal Issues

Adrienne Lam

Overview

Online mental health support is defined broadly as "mental health services and information delivered or enhanced through the internet and related technologies" (Christensen, Griffiths, & Evans, 2002; Shalini & Carol, 2014, p. 24). With barriers such as COVID-19 being a hamper on people's access to mental health sources, this revolutionary system appears to be an ideal substitute. However, this is a platform that has been insufficiently researched. With this flexible online environment for mental health, comes complexities and ethical questions. The platform provides many benefits, such as reducing depression, anxiety, and alcohol use (Lal & Adair, 2014; Robinson, Rodrigues, Fisher, Bailey, & Herrman, 2015; White et al., 2010). Early diagnosis, intervention, more access to mental health professionals, stigma reduction, and equitable access to care for people on low incomes are also proven to transpire (The Royal Australian and New Zealand College of Psychiatrists, 2019). With these advantages, ethical dilemmas are also certain to emerge, including border crossing, confidentiality, privacy, conflicts of interest, and dual relationships.

The lack of in person therapy will swell the amount of self research done on search engines. The ethical dilemmas when using Google are the self diagnosis and self selection for treatment. Bipolar disorder has an assortment of diagnoses, making it more complicated to diagnose. "Externalizing" diagnoses like bipolar disorder may be more favourable to certain people than some "internalizing" diagnoses like personality disorders.

Online Intervention Analysis and the MONACA I Trial

Additionally, in the MONACA I Trial the negative effects of internet based cognitive behavioral therapy interventions for anxiety or depression was analyzed. What was disclosed was 9.3% of participants reporting at least one potentially treatment related adverse event (Rozental et al. 2015). Further analysis concluded that for some people, the intervention generated feelings of anxiety and depression in treatment, while for others it led to continual struggle and frustration caused from the content on the internet platform. Self monitoring in bipolar disorder using randomized, placebo controlled design daily, was focused in the MONACA I trial (Faurholt-Jepsen et al. 2015). It was discovered that when compared to participants in a control condition, participants who received the intervention interestingly had higher depression scores. The authors of the study proposed that the daily observation and hyper consciousness lengthened their already present depression (Berk and Parker 2009).

The Importance of Visual Cues

A chief part in face-to-face therapy is the facial gestures. In an online environment, the interpretation of communication can be altered with non verbal social cues being absent (Childress, 2000; Feijt, de Kort, Bongers, & Ijsselsteijn, 2018). Facial expressions are key to comprehending possible patients' risk of harm that could be forthcoming, or concerning material that clients are attempting to divulge (Feijt et al., 2018; Stern, 2003). This may expose clients to negative social interactions such as cyberbullying, which in turn further deteriorates their mental health (Seabrook, Kern, & Rickard, 2016). Clients could potentially amplify their communication to compensate, overdramatizing to gain external validation and status (Stern, 2003). Riccio (2013) referred to this as 'hyperdramatic interaction'. Of all age groups, young people are most found to be in jeopardy of frequently inflating situations during online interactions (Riccio, 2013).

Cultural awareness plays a part in therapy, and may be relevant depending on the client's age, ethnicity, religious beliefs, or something else. Client's are not liable to reveal any racial or cultural information to their therapist, as it could lead to complaints of implicit or explicit bias. With e-therapy, therapists could miss prudent information that could be caught from a piece of accessory such as a star of David, or a cross necklace, indicating a client's religion.

This is also a portion of the visual cues mentioned earlier; this additional information may or may not be important. Hygiene, clothing, and other physical distinctions may also be valuable to the physician. Therapists are to access a client's wellbeing for their treatment needs, so an accurate assessment is crucial.

Internet Knowledge Insufficiency

A lack of understanding on online exchange can pose a risk as well. Prensky (2001) coined the term 'digital natives' to describe the group of people having grown up during an era where technology was actively integrated in their daily lives, a contrast to 'digital immigrants', the group of people not born in the digital world. This generational divide is representative of the difference in perception of online use and communication. While clinicians may be properly skilled to conduct in-person interactions, they may not have the capacity to properly interpret and manage online interrelations, along with managing subtle online prompts, etc. (Borcsa & Pomini, 2017). Their lack of experience and training can lower their proficiency, leaving their clients safety and wellbeing at a more vulnerable state (Borcsa & Pomini, 2017; Childress, 2000).

Clients and Erratic Appearances

In a virtual environment, clients are prone to inconsistent attendance. "Users participate and then withdraw, then they participate again. They stay or roam and wander off into another space. It is exactly the accentuation of this mobility and speed, of this stop-start process, which gives virtual worlds much of their appeal" (Webb, 2001, p. 587). These intermittent encounters are what network theorists refer to as 'weak ties', and provide individuals knowledge and loose connections, but not the emotional support they need (Granovetter, 1983).

Confidentiality Issues

Onto confidentiality difficulties, boundaries can be crossed in these computer-mediated interactions. In a virtual platform, people tend to lower barriers to social engagement, encouraging clients to be more open and willing to elaborate on sensitive issues like suicidal thoughts and intentions (Notredame et al., 2018; Stern, 2003). While this provides chances for early interventions (Cheng, Chang, & Yip, 2012; Notredame et al., 2018; Rice et al., 2016), it also leaves ethical and confidentiality vulnerabilities. Clinicians find the control of their privacy more unmanageable in the fluidity of online social environments. The risk for personal information breaches increases, therefore it is critically important to inform clients of these potential privacy infringes (Childress, 2000).

For clients undergoing mental health issues and drug and alcohol problems, it can present more difficulties, possibly impairing their judgment. Childress (2000) noted the availability that online support offers, and in this condition create a sense of urgency. Immediate responses are beneficial (Lannin & Scott, 2013), but can raise moral issues, blurring boundaries. The 'off hours' casualty of therapeutic relationships make the differentiation of a boundary more difficult. This lack of clarity is referred to as an "ethical grey zone" from Mishna, Bogo, Root, Sawyer, and Khoury-Kassabri (2012). These situations can result in physician competence uncertainties (Boddy & Dominelli, 2017), or in extreme cases, harassment and stalking (Childress, 2000). In short, the virtual interactive possibilities for privacy conundrums are less explored, and exposes risks for both clients and physicians (Lehavot et al., 2012). More risks are posed in e-therapy. Privacy and confidentiality can be violated with hackers, emails can be sent to the wrong address, or unintentionally exposing any personal information to a recipient (Manhaul-Baugus, 2001). This security breach complicates the computer-mediated situation, a circumstance that can commonly occur. These confidentiality challenges need to come with solutions. A potential solution would be to require passwords when accessing confidential information on their devices. This would allow protection for this information, as passwords make it more difficult to hack into their devices (Heron & J.M., 2010). In the case that the patient receives these e-services in a separate jurisdiction to where they reside such as a different country, there are legal issues including liability and licensing. The challenge is when to act on these data. If social media apps are currently able to predict when someone is at risk for suicide, one may wonder the responsibility e-mental health services have in this (Heron & J.M., 2010). Lastly, another confidentiality issue would be what the information gathered, specifically from behaviour is used for. It has been found that in France, insurers that treat sleep apnoea, no longer fund treatment to those whose computerized monitoring show are 'non-compliant' This shows how some may be excluded from these services if they are found to not comply with computerized monitoring (Heron & J.M., 2010).

Legal Issues

Legal ethical affairs include an online informed consent form. Two options for these signatures are faxed, or signatures in a consent package. These online transactions are considered fully legal as a pen to paper signature. This element includes a further emotional factor in the commitment process. The Digital Signatures Act was formed to "require the adoption and utilization of digital signatures by Federal agencies and to encourage the use of digital signatures in private sector electronic transactions." Moreover, legal sensitivities may arise when jurisdictional questions do (Frankel, 2000; Rosik & Brown, 2001). Getting treated on the internet may cross jurisdictions to a patient's well-being. E-therapy raises questions centering licensure laws in the therapist's state. In the United States. Californian law states that only therapists licensed there may perform their practice online to other residents of California (Frankel, 2000; Rosik & Brown, 2001; Stofle, 1996), although the legal action taken as a consequence towards e-therapists not abiding by the law is not clear. However, it is debatable whether the client's best interest is based on an e-therapist's location, or the state in which the client resides in. Demanding an "every state" licensure may not be the most sensible or functional, such as California's law, because clients may have a difficult time reaching out to therapists that possess the facilities to treat particular mental health disorders, such as trichotillomania. There are alternatives to these restrictive laws, such as e-therapists reviewing if they have the qualifications to treat clients in certain states, with the consideration that the therapist meets the requirement practice laws of the state. This permits them to aid clients without owning a state licensure.

Online Forums

A common online service platform are therapeutic forums. Individuals joining this forum can lend and receive support from other peers with similar experiences. Oftentimes, the admin of these forums are therapists. With the certain arrangement of the site, however, disputes, misuse, or abuse can occur in these, reasoning why ground rules are essential. Terms should be set, as well as a clarification that these forums are not in any way a replacement for professional mental health treatment. Administrators should take action and prohibit those who disobey or violate these rules to establish consequence. The looseness of online forums call for pivotal regulations to ensure that people seeking support are in an ethical and safe environment.

In 2000, many concerns were made over the ethical and legal issues regarding having therapists in the room, discussion groups, and internet technology had just begun to explode. It was said that "…psychotherapy could not be conducted in an ethical manner over the Internet." (Humphreys 2000). If mental health professionals are so unprepared, how can e-mental health thrive with these ethical issues? However, in 2002, 250 locations had started to provision online counselling which was also referred to e-therapy, web-counselling, cyber-therapy, and computer-mediated psychotherapy to name a few (Alleman, 2002). Although they did not predict this to occur, Alleman, Humphreys, Winzelberg, & Klaw addressed some ethical concerns (Alleman, 2002; Humphreys, Winzelberg, & Klaw, 2000). Concerns are important and need to be confronted to evaluate the ethics of e-mental health. They believed that ethical responsibility was not possible for individuals receiving care outside of the jurisdiction they reside. This was because laws concerning privacy and legal issues may apply to one jurisdiction, but not another. If an individual is living in a jurisdiction that has stringent oversight over these ethical issues, but receives care in another jurisdiction, they may not be protected from the same laws which many may not be wary of. The second concern raised was the issue of not being able to see another face-to-face could result in identification issues. A reliable identification process is needed to ensure that one is not impersonated by someone else, as this could undermine the trust in e-mental health, or other e-health care services, so identity is paramount to ensure safety, reliability, and trust. Third, privacy is not guaranteed for typed or recorded communications. Think about the texts you send to your friends, or the phone calls you make to book an appointment. Are they really secure? Do the apps you have respect your privacy, or do they have access to these communications? Just like these interactions we make daily, e-mental health would always provide a privacy challenge.

Guidelines

With the emergence of e-mental health, comes the need for guidelines to be implemented. In Canada, the Canadian Psychological Association created guidelines that inform the provision of psychological services using electronic media. These guidelines are meant to guide the relationship between the client and the psychologist, not for using media to educate or provide resources and other information. There are 4 principles to this guideline: Respect for Dignity of Persons and Peoples, Responsible Caring, Integrity in Relationships, and Responsibility to Society (Canadian Psychological Association, 2017). The first principle involves the providing of information regarding the nature, risks, benefits, and alternative services to the client, as well as other privacy issues they should be concerned about such as interceptions. They need to maximize agreement with their clients, and ensure the best possible security is given to their client, and if this is difficult, something needs to be done to ease their client's concern. The second principle refers to the maximizing benefits and minimizing risks model. Psychologists need to stay up to date with the e-mental health field and literature. If at any time they feel that in person would benefit the client, online service should be switched to in person; e-mental health does not give the maximal benefits and minimal harms to everyone. The third principle involves avoiding conflict of interest. When providing mental health services online, the care provider needs to ensure that the providing these e-services are both convenient and financially advantageous for their clients to serve their unique needs. Lastly, when possible, it is important for psychologists to liability insurance coverage for their e-services, as well as abide by the laws and regulations of their jurisdictions.

Conclusion

In summation, online mental health services can include: the freedom to send and receive messages at any time in the day, having the time to reflect and craft messages to physicians, recorded history of interactions, convenience of scheduling, and the comfort of staying at home. Many individuals struggle with getting dressed, driving, and experience other barriers keeping them from being treated, to which online therapy becomes accessible. People with busy schedules, heavy depression, or therapist interaction anxiety will also find online practices convenient. Unfortunately, this unfamiliarity of a cyberspace can lead to lost messages, security breaches, and many more ethical dilemmas.

Mental health practitioners should keep in mind the disadvantages to maintain a healthy bond with clients, and to take the next steps to prevent them. For therapists, a course of action they can pursue is to ensure clients' data, being mindful of their scope of practice; referring clients when necessary is morally the right thing to do if a physician cannot treat them to the extent they require. Following an ethical obligation to report potential of danger, and forming a strong contact with clients can also avoid an ethical risk. Physicians should practice consent, set clear expectations, and communicate policies accordingly. Above all, clients should be treated with a physician's full ability to strengthen and reach their mental potential.

Detractors and Critics of E-mental Health

Jennifer Pham

Overview

Despite the rising potential of e-mental health services, there remains many concerns and challenges associated with the use of e-mental health resources. Criticism of e-mental health services vary depending on the implementation of these services, which can take numerous forms from simple self-help videos and mood-management apps to online therapy. However, the main concern surrounding e-mental health services is their efficacy as compared to in-person mental health services, such as a traditional in-person therapy session with a therapist or social worker. Additional skepticism comes from the lack of consistency and transparency in guidelines governing user privacy and licensing of therapists on certain e-mental health apps and websites. Although the benefits of introducing e-mental health services come from their potential to increase accessibility and affordability, there remains barriers in terms of technological literacy and insurance coverage. Thus, this chapter will explore the criticism and challenges present in e-mental health resources.

While the development of e-mental health resources have risen in recent years, the efficacy of e-mental health services is still viewed with skepticism when compared to traditional mental health services, namely in-person counselling. Many individuals are more reluctant to use e-mental health services than traditional therapy (Apolinário-Hagen et al., 2018). Surveys on the public's acceptability of e-mental health services often found that participants viewed traditional therapy as significantly more helpful than online services (Apolinário-Hagen et al., 2017). A study, focused on patients with obsessive-compulsive disorder (OCD), found that 75% of patients believed that online therapy would result in small or no improvements in their symptoms (Musiat et al., 2014).

However, the skepticism related to e-mental health services can be attributed to the lack of awareness about what e-mental health services are and how they actually work (Apolinário-Hagen et al., 2017, 2018). In a study on attitudes toward e-mental health services, "e-preferers", those who indicated more experience (15%) with online counseling than "non e-preferers", were more open to using online mental health services (Apolinário-Hagen et al., 2017). For example, "e-preferers" found information websites and Web-based programs without therapist assistance to be more helpful than "non e-preferers", while "non e-preferers" indicated more concerns with e-mental health services (Apolinário-Hagen et al., 2017). Furthermore, the acceptability of e-mental health services vary depending on the type of service. Face-to-face therapy is often used as the point of comparison for e-mental health services (Apolinário-Hagen et al., 2017). Thus, patients might be more open to certain services that incorporate aspects of traditional therapy, such as video-conferencing with a therapist, than self-help treatments.

At the same time, there remains many gaps between online and in-person counselling. One main concern stems from the limited communication through body language with online therapy. Facial expression, tone of voice, moods and body language are all aspects important to in-person counselling as therapists use these cues to interpret and diagnose their patients' mental situation (Moock, 2014). Text-based counselling services completely remove this form of communication. Therapists could only evaluate their patients based on what their patients choose to text them without any additional information from non-verbal cues that are present with in-person counselling. Text-based counselling would also allow the patients to answer at their own pace. The patients are allowed time to "come up" with a response to the therapist rather than immediately respond to what the therapist says. Although a patient does not have to immediately answer their therapist in an in-person counselling session, the patient can react in a non-verbal way and that behaviour can be picked up by a therapist. Even with video-conferencing, micro-expressions are not well conveyed. As work and school were largely moved online during the 2019 coronavirus pandemic, many individuals have expressed feeling "Zoom fatigue" (Wiederhold, 2020). Researchers attributed this phenomenon to the body trying to overcome differences between online and in-person communication (Wiederhold, 2020). Although video-conferencing appears to be in real time, a slight delay still exists in transmitting the participants' response through the screen (Wiederhold, 2020). Video calls also capture mostly the participants' face, and thus, forms of non-verbal communication other than facial expressions are overlooked (Wiederhold, 2020). The lack of non-verbal communication can undermine a therapist's evaluation of their patients. The missing information that would otherwise be available in an in-person therapy session can impair a therapist's diagnostic and psychological assessment process (Stoll et al., 2020).

In addition to body language, online counselling also impedes a therapist's ability to respond in crisis situations. During an in-person session, the therapist is able to assess the patient's conditions and help the patient remain safe. For example, if a patient is experiencing self-harm or suicidal thoughts, the therapist is able to provide more direct assistance to keep their patient safe if they are at the same location. Online therapy, thus, makes it difficult for therapists to respond as they might not be able to obtain or verify the patient's location to send timely help (Stoll et al., 2020). Technological difficulties, such as glitching during video-conferencing, can also interrupt conservations to help calm down the patients. The problem might be worse in the case of text-based therapy where the therapist might not be able to reply immediately. Thus, although e-mental health services transgress the geographical barrier that hinders accessibility to mental health services, the patient and therapist being at different locations can limit the therapist's efforts to help in an emergency or crisis situation (Moock, 2014; Stoll et al., 2020).

The difficulty in maintaining engagement poses another challenge associated with e-mental health services. Scheduling an in-person therapy session involves careful planning, and cancellation of the appointment is not as simple as closing an app. Studies have found that it is difficult to sustain the use of self-guided online treatments (Eysenbach, 2005; Williams et al., 2018). Consistency in treatment is an important aspect of the therapy process and can be disrupted as patients have free range to "log-off" of the e-mental health service when they prefer. However, this challenge can be overcome by incorporating the guide of a therapist. For example, as opposed to self-help resources, patients can set up online appointments with their therapists.

On the other hand, the ability to contact a therapist online can create an illusion that the therapist is always available to the patient. Being able to text and call the therapist from anywhere can make the relationship between the patient and therapist seem more casual (Stoll et al., 2020). For instance, although online therapy allows for flexibility in time and location to communicate with a therapist, the patient or therapist can technically talk while they are on vacation (Stoll et al., 2020), creating a more personal dynamic akin to friendship. The lack of professionalism in the relationship can directly affect the therapy process, such as by leading to biased judgement. Therapists fulfill a specific role that should not be confused with that of a friend or partner.

Criticism of Cross-border Practices

Although e-mental health services increase accessibility by eliminating geographic barriers, the idea that a therapist can practice from anywhere in the world has its own complications. Firstly, the licensing and treatment guidelines differ from one country to another and, in some cases, within a country (Stoll et al., 2020). In the United States, regulations on licensing vary from one state to another (Moock, 2014). Thus, one of the main issues with online therapy is in how it can be regulated. There are currently no legal committees or organizations that provide clear guidelines on how cross-border practice should be conducted (Stoll et al., 2020). The lack of international regulation becomes problematic when a concern is raised or a violation in practice occurs. The case could be judged according to licensing and treatment guidelines within the therapist's or the patient's location; thus, differences in these guidelines could change the outcome of the case and the person who should take responsibility (Stoll et al., 2020). The issues regarding licensing are further complicated by the danger of fraud. The identity of the therapist, and even the patient, may be difficult to verify online and can lead to scenarios where a therapist is practicing without proper licensing, or a therapist treating a minor without consent of a parent or guardian (Stoll et al., 2020). Thus, the lack of international regulations and prevalence of fraud can easily lead to unethical practices with online therapy .

Another issue that can arise with online therapy is the lack of training on the therapist's part on international practices. The therapist might not be aware of treatment guidelines in the patient's jurisdiction (Stoll et al., 2020), which can lead to differences in expectations of how the treatment is conducted. Online therapy might also need to overcome culture differences if the therapist and patients are in different countries (Stoll et al., 2020). Culture can influence behaviour and being aware of the cultural differences may help in the process of therapy. Since cultural differences may still exist in treating a patient from the same country, being in different countries can add on another layer to this barrier.

Costs and Insurance

The cost of e-mental health services vary depending on the type of service and service provider. Overall, e-mental health services are often praised to be more cost-effective than in-person therapy. While in-person therapy can cost hundreds of dollars, online therapy is seen as a better alternative with apps such as Betterhelp, which charges $65-80 USD per week (Hoy & Lee, 2021), and Talkspace, which charges $260-396 USD per month (Talkspace, 2021). However, considering the relatively new rise of e-mental health services, many insurance policies do not provide coverage for online therapy (Moock, 2014). Therefore, costs would have to be paid out of pocket without any reimbursement (Moock, 2014).

Privacy

As with licensing, there seems to be a lack of regulation when it comes to patient's privacy and confidentiality (Marshall et al., 2020; Stoll et al., 2020). In order to ensure privacy for the patient, information provided on e-mental health services needs to be encrypted. Privacy legislation may also differ from one country to another. In addition, patients who share a living space with other individuals may not be able to share their information privately. In this case, patients might feel uncomfortable and less inclined to share very personal information. Thus, remote therapy not only poses a privacy challenge to providers in terms of securely storing patients' personal data but also to patients in terms of sharing personal information.

App Developers Guidelines

The lack of regulation can also make it difficult to give e-mental health resource designers and developers guidelines that would follow those of regulatory agencies such as the Food and Drug Administration, the Federal Joint Committee, NICE, Therapeutic Goods Administration and Medsafe (Moock, 2014). Policies regarding licensing and privacy may differ from one service provider to another and differ from traditional practice regulation. For example, the terms and conditions of Betterhelp, an online therapy service, state: "We do not control the quality of the Counselor Services and we do not determine whether any Counselor is qualified to provide any specific service as well as whether a Counselor is categorized correctly or matched correctly to you" (Lorenz, 2018). The terms also include that the "Counselor Services are not a complete substitute for a face-to-face examination and/or session by a licensed qualified professional" (Lorenz, 2018). Thus, e-mental health service users need to be careful of the terms of their service providers.

Concerns with Technological Usage

The reliance on technology creates an accessibility barrier for e-mental health services. Certain services, such as online therapy, may require proper equipment with a camera or webcam and a microphone, not just any device. Also, participants would often require a stable Internet connection. However, not everyone is able to afford such equipment and Internet access. According to a study conducted in 2019, there is a "digital divide" between socioeconomic groups, where 95% of those in the higher socioeconomic group own a smartphone while only 71% of those in the lower socioeconomic group own a smartphone (Marshall et al., 2020). Slow internet speeds can affect the quality of video-conferences, access to videos and websites, etc. Technical difficulties can potentially lead to disruptions or termination of an online therapy session. Such situations may be difficult to handle and can lead to frustrations on both parts (Stoll et al., 2020). While individuals can access equipment and the Internet from places other than their homes, privacy concern arises. Public areas such as libraries cannot ensure user's privacy and confidentiality (Williams et al., 2018).

Furthermore, technological literacy places another accessibility barrier for e-mental health services. In order to go on apps and websites and access the Internet, patients need to have some experience with technology. However, some consumers, especially older consumers, may lack the skills to properly use technology (Williams et al., 2018). The cognitive capacity of the patient may also pose another challenge in using technology (Williams et al., 2018). The concern with technology literacy does not only apply to patients but therapists as well. Therapists might not have received training in using online resources, or were given enough time to understand how these resources work. However, the issue with technological literacy may differ from one therapist to another as younger therapists might be more experienced with e-resources than older therapists (Marshall et al., 2020). Nonetheless, technological literacy challenges the accessibility of e-mental health services.

The use of technology in psychotherapy is another point of concern. In recent years, social media has often been criticized for being linked to mental health issues (Moock, 2014). As aforementioned, online communication misses many facets of in-person communication such as tone and body language.

Online communication lacks the physicality of human-to-human interactions, and can lead to feelings of disconnectedness. A study on computerized cognitive behavioural therapy (cCBT) found that patients with severe symptoms of depression generally indicated negative feelings toward cCBT (Musiat et al., 2014). The study also proposed that computerized treatments can increase social isolation (Musiat et al., 2014). Thus, the use of e-mental health services have been suggested as an addition to traditional therapy rather than a substitute for it.

Language Barrier

Lack of proficiency in English creates a challenge to using technology, and in turn, e-mental health services. Since many e-mental health apps and websites are in English, non-English speakers are less likely to access those resources (Reyes et al., 2018). Although this issue exists with in-person therapy, therapist offices might be able to offer translating services to the patients. However, the same solution can not be applied to situations where patients need help understanding the instructions to set up an app or access a website. This language barrier adds on another layer to problems with accessibility of e-mental health services.

Therapist Guided E-Mental Health Services

As suggested above, e-mental health services can be used along with traditional therapy with a therapist rather than a substitute to in-person services. A study on acceptability of e-mental health services reported that participants find therapist-assisted treatments, whether online or in-person, as more helpful than unguided treatments (Apolinário-Hagen et al., 2017). Another study found that therapists' participation in e-mental health services alongside patients increased engagement and eased navigation of the sites used (Williams et al., 2018). Thus, the degree of assistance provided by the therapist also influences patients' attitude and experience with e-mental health services.

May Not Be Applicable to All Forms of Mental Disorders

Even though guided services seem to provide a balance between e-mental health resources and traditional therapy services, the use of e-mental health services overall may not be compatible for all mental disorders. Studies find that, while online therapy may be appropriate for mild to moderate mental health disorders, it may not be suitable at all for more severe disorders (Stoll et al., 2020). For example, those with psychiatric disorders may be recommended for online psychotherapy if they present a danger to themselves or others (Stoll et al., 2020).

Conclusion

E-mental health services seemingly provide a good alternative to traditional in-person therapy by eliminating certain accessibility and cost barriers. However, these services have their own set of disadvantages and concerns. E-mental health services are still not able to replace certain facets of in-person therapy. The lack of regulation with remote mental health services presents many problems in licensing, privacy and costs. The use of technology creates other accessibility barriers not present in traditional therapy. Last but not least, e-mental health services may not be appropriate for all types and degrees of mental health disorders. Thus, criticism and concerns with e-mental health services should continue to be addressed and explored to help improve the quality of care for all patients.

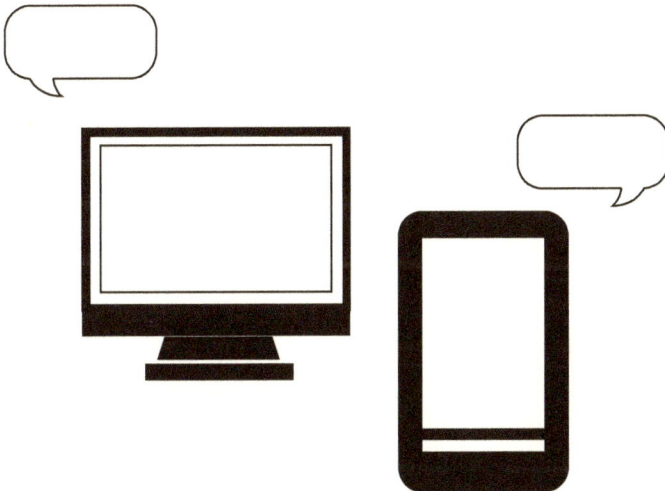

How Different Cultures View E-mental Health

Abeer Ansari

Culture has a profound impact on the perception of mental health, mental illness and mental health services (Satcher, 2001). There exists a lot of diversity in ideas and personal experiences across cultures and thus different cultures view mental health struggles differently which also shakes how they view the interventions and treatment for poor mental health. It is important for one to understand how a culture perceives mental health struggles in order to create a treatment plan that best suits the values and approach of that specific cultural group (Satcher, 2001). Since mental health struggles are common all around the world, the different disorders and symptoms are all organized in the Diagnostic and Statistical Manual of Mental Disorders which is a tool used by clinicians from all around the world, irrespective of their culture, to make a diagnosis and determine treatments for common disorders. However, there also exists mental health struggles and symptoms that are specific to a single culture and this specification requires a thorough understanding of that culture's traditions and values and how it perceives mental health. A concept that is crucial to understanding when analysing cross cultural mental health is the concept of culture-bound syndromes (Satcher, 2001).

141

These are a group of symptoms that tend to be relevant in some cultural societies more than others. For example, if a culture has a tradition of having its women stay in isolation during pregnancy while other cultures do not practice this tradition, then one might expect to see mental health related symptoms of pregnancy related depression that is more prevalent in that specific culture. In addition to culture-bound syndromes, cultures also include whether or not people will seek treatment for their mental illness and the types of treatment that they will seek out. Moreover, the social environment of an individual contributes to shaping their perception and the meaning they assign to their personal struggles all of which has a direct impact on the type of coping mechanisms and resources they look out for (Satcher, 2001).

As discussed in earlier chapters, one strong benefit of e-mental health treatment services is the fact that they have the potential of reaching people outside their immediate geographical location which means that it is very likely to be paired with a clinician who belongs to a different culture than the patient themselves (Aggarwal, 2012). It is important to note that the cultural background of the clinician, especially when accessing e-mental health services, plays an important role in the delivery and quality of care. This chapter will further discuss how differences in the culture of the health care provider and patient impacts how people of certain cultures will perceive the idea of using e-mental health especially in the context of cross cultural services and resources

(Aggarwal, 2012). Finally, this chapter will analyze the differences that exist between South Asian and Western cultures when accessing e-mental health services.

Importance of the culture of the patient

There are various different ways a culture and social environment affect numerous factors that are important for a struggling patient who is seeking out help (Satcher, 2001). The presentation of symptoms, or how a patient describes their symptoms is highly influenced by culture. In understanding this idea, it is important to know the two different categories of symptoms: somatic symptoms and emotional symptoms. Somatic symptoms refer to physical symptoms that affect one's health such as headaches or abdominal pain versus emotional symptoms which may include feelings of excessive sadness or stress. Patients who belong to an Asian culture are more comfortable in reporting their somatic symptoms while avoiding conversations about their emotional symptoms (Satcher, 2001). A research study highlighted that Asian patients only presented their physical symptoms to their clinician while they later resorted in self report scales that they indeed did experience emotional symptoms as well but chose not to talk about them with their health care provider (Aggarwal, 2012). This illustrates the cultural differences that exist when it comes to the symptoms reported by patients.

Culture also influences how the patient perceives their mental health struggles and symptoms. There are some cultures in which people will associate their mental health struggles to tests from God and thus will prefer seeing a spiritual healer or pastoral. In some cases, they would refrain from seeking help while cultures that perceive mental health struggles as a medical illness might be more likely to reach out to medical professionals such as a primary health care provider or mental health specialist (Aggarwal, 2012). It is important to note that the type of resource individuals reach out to can have. A huge impact on the quality of their life and lack of understanding or high level of stigma can make people of certain cultures avoid reaching out for help which can lead to further distress, physical and mental disability and the possibility of suicide.

The family system tends to be perceived as a strong support system however, culture influences the family dynamic and familial factors of support (Satcher, 2001). Family factors have the potential of protecting an individual from mental health struggles while also having the potential of contributing towards the development of a mental health struggle or mental illness. For example, a supportive family that respects an individual's personal boundaries and promotes the idea of building trust and comfort within the family unit is linked with better mental health outcomes. However, family units can also be very toxic as in the case of domestic abuse, child abuse and neglect. The likelihood of a family unit serving as a protective factor or as a risk varies across cultural and ethnic groups (Satcher, 2001).

Culture also plays a huge role in the development of coping mechanisms (Satcher, 2001). Coping mechanisms are skills and tools people use to cope with their problems and to navigate their way out of challenging and stressful situations. For example, South Asians believe that avoidance disorder is better than confrontation and thus they tend not to focus on their problems and cope by distracting themselves in order to avoid problematic aspects of their life as they believe that suppression is better than expression of feelings and concerns (Aggarwal, 2012). While on the other hand, African Americans are more likely to face their problems head on, they believe that actively dealing with problems is much more effective than avoiding them. Furthermore, African Americans, when comforted to White people, are more likely to handle their problems on their own and rely on spiritual healers when seeking help (Blumenfield, 2020). It is important to understand these culture laws differences when analyzing the use of e-mental health services in different cultures because those e-mental health resources must take into account the difference in coping mechanisms when creating a treatment and intervention plan in order to emerge that patients received culturally appropriate care (Satcher, 2001).

Finally cultural values and factors are a strong determining factor in treatment seeking behaviour and approach of people (Satcher, 2001). There are variations in the likelihood of seeking treatment and the choice of clinician across different cultures. For example, those who belong to racial and ethnicity minority groups are less likely to reach out for help when compared to white people living in the United States. Moreover, minority groups are more likely to delay the process aid seeking out for help and only really reach out when their symptoms have significantly worsened. Moreover, research has indicated that even when these minority groups reach out for help, they tend to go to primary care physicians instead of mental health specialists even when they are aware of their mental illness. Studies of African Americans seeking out help have shown that they tend to prefer a clinician who is from the same cultural and ethnic background as them (Satcher, 2001). This finding enhances our understanding as to how African Americans and people of other minority groups may use e-mental health services especially when it has the potential of connecting patients and clinicians from different cultures. One common and strong factor that will help explain the difference in treatment seeking behaviour across cultures is the idea of mistrust. Mistrust has been deemed a significant barrier in accessing mental health services especially when it comes to racial and ethnic minority groups. In a Epidemiological Catchment Area study, researchers obtained survey responses from African Americans and Whites in regards to mental health related treatments (Satcher, 2001). The results conveyed that African Americans who were suffering from severe depression opted out from getting hospitalized due to their fear of being treated in a hospital. This mistrust arises due to historical persecution and discrimination against certain curtural and ethnic groups. It is important to understand this rather crucial factor and increase the

146

availability of practitioners who belong to minority groups and grant them training and access to e-mental health platforms so they can deliver quality, trustful care and bridge the gap that exists within the delivery of equitable mental health care (Satcher, 2001).

Previous chapters have highlighted the importance and benefits of e-mental health, while this chapter has discussed the differences in cultures when it comes to perceiving mental health struggles and treatments. Therefore, it is now crucial to discuss the importance of making internet based interventions adaptable for different cultural and ethnic backgrounds in order to enhance the quality and effectiveness of psychological care.

Researchers performed a systematic literature review using popular databases including PsycINFO, MEDLINE, WoS, CENTRAL and Embase (Spanhel, 2020). Their literature review focused on "mental disorders", "Internet and Mobile-Based Interventions", and "cultural adaptation." The goal was to determine the effectiveness of internet based treatment when it was tailored to be culturally appropriate by studying patient outcomes for those treatments (Spanhel, 2020). Most internet and mobile based interventions are catered towards those fluent in the English language and have access to the latest technological interfaces. However, the cultural adaptation of these e-mental health services through the conversation of language and cultural barriers as well as the patient's personal values and morals has been associated with enhancing the effectiveness of these Internet and mobile based psychological treatments (Spanhel, 2020).

E-mental Health and Cultural Adaptation

Cross cultural patient care is when care is delivered by a health care provider who belongs to a cultural background different from that of the patient's (Mucic, 2016). Factors that prevent individuals from seeking desired care include the long geographical distances, cultural and religious differences, language barriers that prevent effective communication and understanding. To overcome some of these challenges, e-mental health resources come in handy as they may provide language specific resources and culturally specific services. Research has shown that the use of interpreters during therapy and other psychological treatments takes away from the direct connection that would otherwise be strong between the health care provider and the patient (Mucic, 2016). Information usually gets lost between translation and in some cultures, there might be lack of words to explain certain emotions. Moreover, this chapter has earlier discussed other significant factors that impact one's mental health and the likelihood of them receiving effective treatment and how those factors differ across cultures. The good news is that e-mental health services and applications bridge the cultural and communication gap by matching patients with mental health professionals whose profile indicates that they belong to the same cultural background (Mucic, 2016). This is a huge advancement in the field of mental health care since it will allow people who would have otherwise not reached out for help to now feel safe and confident in accessing mental health services (Mucic, 2016). After being "matched" with the clinicians, patients do not have to travel long distances to receive the support that they need. While e-mental health services limit the real time experience, the fact that more people are not able to access care is definitely a benefit that outweighs the limitations (Mucic, 2016).

It is also proposed that the clinicians attitude towards using e-mental health services is also a strong determining factor as to how effective the treatment and intervention would be (Mucic, 2016). Clinicians who tend to have a positive and promising outlook about e-mental health services tend to increase the positive experience of both the clinician and patient. Therefore, it is important to educate clinicians about the following factors that are important for people who belong to different cultures and thus they should opt out to use e-mental health services for the sake of their patients when needed. These will help them realize the promising results that can be achieved through virtual platforms and increase their positive perception about delivering quality care online (Mucic, 2016). Clinicians who are either from the same background as their patient or from a different background must understand the following cultural implications in order to develop an appreciation of e-mental health services and enhance their care: the first concept is stereotyping. When interacting with individuals from a different culture, stereotyping becomes very easy and often time is done unconsciously but it can have a huge impact on the relationship that is being established between the healthcare provider and the patient. Hence, it is best to avoid engaging in ethnocentric approaches that arise due to comparing one's own culture to someone else's. It is important to understand that certain cultures have individualistic values while other cultures may be more interdependent. This can also impact treatment since people from individualistic cultures may be willing to maintain a stronger sense of confidentiality and autonomy throughout the treatment process while those who have interdependent values may prefer to have a larger support system accompany them during their treatment process (Aggarwal, 2012). These differences are important to understand for two main reasons: to prepare clinicians of different backgrounds as they use e-mental health services to deliver care so they can orient themselves to the wide range of diverse patient populations. The second reason is for clinicians of the same cultural backgrounds as their patients to develop an understanding as to how important these e-mental health services are for the patient to receive effective care and so they should appreciate the availability of these services and view it from a positive outlook (Mucic, 2016).

In conclusion, e-mental health services have played a huge role in bridging the cultural and ethnic gap that prevented many people from receiving the care that they needed. While these services do limit direct human contact and might be fairly new to some societies, the fact that it can connect patients to clinicians of their own cultural background regardless of their location and cost associated with travelling is an advantage that will help decrease the stigma and promote mental well-being across cultures.

Future Technologies for E-mental Health

Aaliyah Mulla

Overview

As technological advances continue to grow, so does the breadth of their applications. While mental health services were once offered primarily in an in-person format, they have been increasingly offered in a wider range of mediums, as discussed in previous chapters. One of the first applications of e-mental health was the use of suicide hotlines, which are now used to address other mental-health-related crises as well. Stemming from hotlines was the adoption of chat-based counselling, and the possibilities of e-mental health services have only expanded since.

Three Main Categories of Future Technologies

Currently, there appears to be three broad categories of future technologies needed to advance the field of e-mental health. First, high-quality, creative technology to offer a wide range of mental health services. Second, technology to develop the digital infrastructure needed for widespread adoption of such technology, and third, technology to collect data from large populations that can be used to inform the creation of new services.

153

The first category is arguably the most expansive and exciting of the three, with seemingly endless possibilities. This type of technology includes conventional phone-based and chat-based counselling, and virtual therapy using videoconferencing software. As technology continues to evolve and the demand for e-mental health services increases, more creative approaches are emerging.

Moving beyond traditional weekly appointments with a therapist, some companies have developed mobile apps and cultivated virtual community spaces for people to seek help as and when they need it. Some of these services are meant for temporary aid and they connect patients with counselors, while others include long-term treatment plans with qualified clinicians.

One of the first examples of such a service is called eheadspace (Grainger and Barnes, 2020). This platform offers Australian youth temporary help through a number of services, including the ability to connect with qualified mental health professionals — all free of charge. The platform also offers chat-based group therapy, where youth can connect with peers to explore topics together with the guidance of a professional. Moreover, it has a multitude of resources covering a range of topics, from addiction to job-searching. In order for youth to identify and organise the resources that are most relevant to them, eheadspace has a platform for them to assemble their own mental health toolkits, called, "spaces". Unfortunately, eheadspace is only available in Australia, but it is likely that with growing demand and awareness, similar services will be adopted elsewhere.

For now, Canada offers a number of other e-mental health services — some free and some which require payments (Humi Team, 2020). For instance, Talkspace and BetterHelp both offer flexible e-therapy arrangements with qualified therapists and psychiatrists. These are alternatives to face-to-face therapy and allow patients to access therapists through video calls as well as over chats. Some platforms, such as InkBlot, Big Whitewall, and the Centre For Interactive Mental Health Solutions (CIMHS) offer self-guided services (Humi Team, 2020).

Another exciting area of e-mental health is the use of virtual reality (VR) in therapy (Martin, 2019). So far, VR has been used primarily in exposure therapy, which is used to treat anxiety disorders such as phobias (Maples-Keller et.al, 2017). Traditionally, this type of therapy involves exposing a patient to situations or objects that typically elicit the anxiety response (APA, 2017). For instance, if a person has arachnophobia — a fear of spiders — they might first be exposed to pictures of spiders, then toy spiders, and eventually real spiders. This same exposure can be performed using virtual reality instead of physical exposure, which is far more convenient and often the only practical way to conduct such therapy for certain phobias, such as a fear of heights (APA, 2017).

More recently, professionals have been looking into using virtual reality to help diagnose disorders such as autism spectrum disorder (ASD), attention deficit hyperactivity disorder (ADHD), schizophrenia, and even Alzheimer's disease (Martin, 2019). These applications will be discussed in more detail later in this chapter.

With the development of increasingly sophisticated artificial intelligence (AI), people have been looking into self-guided virtual reality-based treatments, similar to self-help books (Martin, 2019). This would involve having patients find applications or software and work through exposure therapy themselves, with a virtual, AI therapist to guide them through the process, instead of undergoing this therapy in-person during a regular therapy session (Martin, 2019). This could offer incredible convenience and make therapy more accessible for those living in remote areas. It would likely also be more affordable. A typical therapy session can cost anywhere from $60-$240 per hour (Gusinksy, 2019). In contrast, it is likely that after the initial costs of developing the AI software, costs associated with maintaining such a service would be minimal. However, this type of technology would need to be crafted carefully to ensure the safety and wellbeing of patients. When patients undergo exposure therapy in-person, therapists are able to monitor their reactions, as well as their vitals, such as heart rate and breathing, to prevent the therapy from getting too overwhelming (Martin, 2019). In a self-guided format, creative approaches would be needed to ensure that patients know when to modify or cut-short an exposure session to avoid an overly strong anxiety response.

One way this could be done is by including a sensor within the VR technology to monitor a patient's vitals. This could be similar to a wearable health or fitness tracker (such as a Fitbit, for instance), which could provide statistics about heart rate, breathing, and other vitals. Connecting a monitor of this sort with an AI-based therapist would allow the AI to recognise when a patient is getting overwhelmed, and thereby modify or end an exposure session when needed. In addition to this, if patients consult with a certified clinician before commencing self-guided therapy of this sort, they can work with a clinician to establish safe parameters based on their individual baselines. These can then be inputted into the AI so that all patients have a program tailored specifically for them. After the initial consultation, the patient would be better prepared to work through the remote therapy on their own.

Wearable health or fitness trackers can also have applications beyond self-guided exposure therapy. Apps and devices that monitor vitals such as heart rate, breathing, and even brain waves, already exist to help people monitor their symptoms (OneMindPsyberGuide, n.d.). For instance, MyBivy is an app that collects information about body rhythms during sleep. It is used by veterans experiencing post-traumatic stress disorder (PTSD) to help them and their veterans affairs (VA) doctors better understand their sleep patterns

(OneMindPsyberGuide, n.d.). Information about sleep patterns can be invaluable in treating the incapacitating night terrors associated with PTSD — also known as nightmare disorder — which can have devastating impacts on a person's quality of life. Information collected by a smartwatch, equipped with a heart rate monitor, is sent to the app and can then be made available to VA doctors (OneMindPsyberGuide, n.d.). Most impressively, the app can also be programmed to disrupt nightmares (Marill, 2020). When the monitor senses that a person is experiencing symptoms that signal the beginning of a nightmare, it can send vibrations through the smartwatch to disturb sleep just enough to prevent the nightmare from progressing, without actually waking the user (Marill, 2020). Since its inception by youth at a hackathon, MyBivy has been rebranded to NightWear (Marill, 2020). NightWare is currently available in a limited capacity, by prescription only, primarily for war veterans (NightWare, 2020). It is still under the process of clinical trials, after which it will likely become more widely available to the general public (Nightware, 2015).

Some companies, such as Toronto-based Awake Labs, are working on applications of similar sensors to help patients manage and monitor stress levels on a day-to-day basis (O'Hara, 2019). This can be useful for many people, including those with intellectual disabilities who may experience stress more often than most, and who may have a hard time communicating their feelings to caregivers (Palmer, 2020). This technology involves sensors built into a smartwatch which send information about heart rate to an app, where caregivers or self-advocates can access the data (Palmer, 2020).

Other services, such as Careware, measure other metrics in addition to heart rate, such as accelerometer data and electrodermal activity (EDA) (Debard et.al, 2020). Accelerometers measure a person's movement (Medical Alert Advice, n.d.), while electrodermal activity is another term for galvanic skin response (GSR) (Benedek and Kaernbach, 2010). Essentially, EDA measures tiny changes in sweat which indicate when a person is stressed (Critchley and Nagai, 2013). Heart rate, on the other hand, is typically measured using blood volume pulse (BVP), which is essentially the amount of blood flowing through a certain area — such as a fingertip or earlobe — at a certain time (Jones, 2018). Since the heart's primary responsibility is to pump blood through the body, monitoring changes in blood volume is a good indication of heart activity.

These measures can send input to an app which can then present the data in a way that is easily accessible to patients and their clinicians or caregivers (Debard et.al, 2020). Over time, algorithms built into the app software can calculate a user's baseline levels of the measures, including heart rate variability — the amount that a person's heart rate typically fluctuates (Debard et.al, 2020). The app can then compare baseline levels with real-time data to determine if levels are out of the ordinary, which may signal the beginning of a mental health crisis. Some devices even measure movement patterns and social interactions, vocal tone and speed, and behaviour at different times of day (NIMH, 2019). Significant changes in any of these measures may signal the onset of a mood episode, such as mania, depression, or psychosis (NIMH, 2019). Early detection of these episodes can help prevent them from escalating to a level that would put a person in crisis by warning people to get help before symptoms worsen (NIMH, 2019). Data like this can also be compared with geotracking or self-report measures so that users become aware of the circumstances that commonly trigger anxiety or mood episodes, which can provide insight into why they experience these symptoms and ultimately help them avoid or control their triggers (Grainger and Barnes, 2020).

Intriguingly, there are even some technologies that monitor brain waves, such as Muse (OneMindPsyberGuide, n.d.). Muse is a sleek headband that measures the electrical activity of the brain, and is used to help people manage their stress levels and improve the quality of their meditation (Knable, 2015). It does so by sending information about brain activity to a mobile app, which then sends feedback back to the user in the form of natural weather sounds (Muse, n.d.). Users hear peaceful weather when they are calm, and louder, more violent weather (such as a storm) when they are not (Muse, n.d.). This helps users identify when their brain is overactive during meditation, motivating them to calm down and then remain in a calm state. Other companies, such as Brainbot, are working on their own products similar to Muse, so it is likely that this technology will be more widely available in the future

(Knable, 2015). Like many e-mental health technologies, Muse does not use brand-new technology, but has adapted pre-existing technology into a portable, more user-friendly format. The actual sensor in the headband is essentially an electroencephalogram machine (EEG), which are machines that are used frequently in clinical settings to measure and monitor brain activity (Muse, n.d.). In fact, even the idea of providing feedback to a patient about their brain activity during meditation is a technique, called neurofeedback, that has been used in therapy sessions for quite some time (Knable, 2015). Muse is unique in that it is far more cost effective and convenient, as it allows people to use it regularly in the comfort of their own home without the need for official therapy sessions (Knable, 2015).

In general, wearables are currently being developed either as watches, headbands, rings, clothing patches, or even tattoos (Grainger and Barnes, 2020). However, one company has taken the idea of wearables to the next level. Otsuka Pharmaceutical has developed a pill with embedded sensors, called Abilify MyCite, which provides information about drug usage when swallowed (Grainger and Barnes, 2020). This can be useful for patients with mental illnesses like schizophrenia, bipolar disorder, or major depressive disorder, who may have difficulty remembering if and when they have taken their medications (Abilify MyCite, n.d.). Currently, the pill contains a minuscule sensor, which is connected to a wearable patch, which sends information to the Abilify MyCite app (Abilify MyCite, n.d.). The app then presents data about whether a patient has taken their medications, and allows patients to input data about their mood (Abilify MyCite, n.d.). This technology sounds exciting, but it is still in relatively early stages when it comes to determining its usefulness, safety, and effectiveness. The company website lists a plethora of potential side effects, many of which are quite serious. Moreover, since the technology is still in the process of being thoroughly tested, it remains unclear if it can actually help improve the likelihood of patients taking their medications (Abilify MyCite, n.d.). Nevertheless, the idea of ingestible sensors is one that, with time and creativity, can potentially be adapted for a wide range of uses.

Technology for Data Collection and Diagnostic Purposes

In addition to having therapeutic benefits, many e-mental health technologies can be used for data collection and diagnostic purposes.

Wearable sensors can collect information about stress levels in individuals to help professionals identify specific populations where poor mental health may be more prevalent. This would signal that more services need to be made available in those specific locations, or that certain interventions need to take place to control factors that may be contributing to poor mental health (Jorm et al., 2013). The portability and convenience of wearables makes it easier for large trials to be conducted to obtain substantive datasets from large sample groups. This would make it easier to establish accurate baselines for vitals such as heart rate and galvanic skin response, and facilitate a better understanding of what variation in these vitals may look like when people experience symptoms of mental illnesses. It also helps researchers understand which interventions work best for specific mental illnesses or specific social groups (Jorm et al., 2013). Data collected in this manner could also be compared to existing health records or even genome sequences in order to better understand individual differences (Jorm et al., 2013). With the influx of such large amounts of data, new approaches may be needed to store, analyse, and interpret this data securely and effectively (Jorm et al., 2013).

As discussed earlier in this chapter, virtual reality is also being used to develop e-mental health treatments. The biggest advantage of VR is that it allows people to do things that would normally be physically impractical or impossible. For instance, Alzheimer's disease is characterised by severe memory deficits, usually affecting elderly people as opposed to young people. However, it also involves impairments in spatial navigation. Typically, spatial navigation can be difficult to measure using traditional tests, and impractical to measure using more immersive techniques, such as asking a patient to navigate their way from one location to another (Martin, 2019). In contrast, VR presents a unique, practical way to test spatial navigation in a controlled environment. By using VR to test for navigational impairment, clinicians can diagnose Alzheimer's patients early, which can lead to better treatment (Martin, 2019).

VR can also be used to diagnose conditions such as autism, attention-deficit hyperactivity disorder (ADHD), and schizophrenia (Martin, 2019). These diagnoses often rely on self-report or interview-based measures, which can lack standardisation (Martin, 2019). In contrast, VR allows for all patients to be given the same test, making diagnoses more objective (Martin, 2019).

Technology to Develop Digital Infrastructure for Widespread Adoption of E-mental Health

While all of these innovative technologies are exciting, they inevitably raise concerns about regulation and quality control, accessibility, and security.

E-mental health is a relatively new field, and has only recently gained increasing popularity (Strudwick et.al, 2020). As such, it can be challenging to ensure new treatments and technology are universally accepted by clinicians and insurance companies (Strudwick et.al, 2020). The novelty of the field, paired with the rapid technological advances that constitute it and the widespread availability of such technology can pose jurisdictional challenges when it comes to policy and insurance claims. In order to resolve these challenges, new structures may be needed to ensure that treatments are covered by insurance plans even if they stray from typical methods. Since e-mental health technologies can usually be accessed from anywhere in the world, international solutions may need to be created to ensure people are covered even when accessing services based abroad. Similarly, innovative funding options may need to be formed to ensure that companies can afford to service patients internationally (Jorm et.al, 2013). For instance, Australia was one of the first countries to adopt e-mental health therapies, so it was challenging at first for them to fund their services when their funding came from the Australian government, but their services were being used by people around the world (Jorm et.al, 2013).

Another problem with technology moving so quickly is that regulations and quality control have not always kept up with the fast pace. This has led to many apps and virtual therapy options being available without evidence that they are effective, which can make it very challenging to decide which, if any, virtual treatment options are best suited to a given individual (NIMH, 2019). So far, sites like One Mind PsyberGuide are good resources to consult, as they provide ratings of a services' credibility, user experience, and transparency. However, there are many services that have simply not yet been tested, and a lack of data does not necessarily mean a service is not effective. For this reason, it is important that the research surrounding e-mental health technologies be better funded.

In some cases, research and testing takes too long to be practical, as technology is moving so quickly that software may become outdated by the time sufficient tests have been conducted (NIMH, 2019). The nature of these situations may require novel approaches to quality control. For instance, NightWear, discussed earlier in this chapter, was approved for accelerated testing because the FDA recognised the importance that it be made available as soon as possible to prevent PTSD symptoms from becoming incapacitating or even life-threatening (Marill, 2020). Similar measures may need to be taken for other services to ensure they can be used by patients in a timely manner. Having standardised quality control regulations can help ensure people spend their time and money wisely on treatments that are most effective for them, and should make it easier to ensure therapies are covered by insurance plans.

Robust technology is also needed to ensure the data of users are completely protected, as e-mental health services often collect a lot of sensitive personal information. Software may need to be developed to ensure applications are collecting and storing information in a manner that is protected from attempts to use the data in a malicious manner.

Along with being secure and supported by evidence, e-mental health services need to be user-friendly (NIMH, 2019). This could involve interactive or even game-like approaches (NIMH, 2019). The easier and more enjoyable these services are to use and navigate, the more effective they will be in treating mental health disorders and facilitating the health and wellbeing of users.

All of these new approaches will likely lead to a change in the types of professions required in the field of mental health (Jorm et.al, 2013). It may be necessary to have people who have been specifically trained in remote counseling, or who have been trained to navigate specific software in addition to their typical therapeutic duties. Some professions may be created specifically to support people through self-guided therapy (Jorm et.al, 2013). Regardless, as is the case for many fields, the field of mental health will likely see increasing opportunities for remote and flexible work schedules.

Conclusion

Overall, the field of e-mental health looks to have a promising future. Many technologies exist already, with a great deal more on the brink of being fully developed for widespread adoption. As these technologies become more easily accessible, it is likely that mental health services will become as ubiquitous as other health services. It is entirely plausible that mental-health check-ins will become as common as dental appointments, meditation exercises as frequent as teeth brushing, and heart rate monitors as common an indicator of stress as eye bags are of fatigue.

References

Background of E-mental Health

About Walk Along. (n.d.). https://walkalong.ca/about-us/general.

Bartram, M. (2012). *Changing directions, changing lives: the mental health strategy for Canada.*
Mental Health Commission of Canada.

Benefits of e-mental health treatments and interventions.
RANZCP. (2019).
https://www.ranzcp.org/news-policy/policy-and-advocacy/position-statements/benefits-e-mental-health-treatments-interventions#:~:text=Telepsychiatry%20services%20can%20p
rovide%20more,who%20are%20in%20most%20need.

Ben-Zeev, D., Brenner, C. J., Begale, M., Duffecy, J., Mohr, D. C., & Mueser, K. T. (2014).
Feasibility, acceptability, and preliminary efficacy of a smartphone intervention for
schizophrenia. *Schizophrenia bulletin, 40*(6), 1244–1253.
https://doi.org/10.1093/schbul/sbu033.

Big Data. big data - what is big data and how is it applied to healthcare? (n.d.).
https://innovatemedtec.com/digital-health/big-data.

Bolton, P. (2019). *Global mental health and psychotherapy: Importance of task-shifting and a* *systematic approach to adaptation.* In D. J. Stein, J. K. Bass, & S. G. Hofmann (Eds.), *Global mental health and psychotherapy: Adapting psychotherapy for low- and* *middle-income countries* (p. 11–24). Elsevier Academic Press. https://doi.org/10.1016/B978-0-12-814932-4.00001-X

Canadian Digital Health Survey. (2020) Canada Health Infoway. Retrieved from: www.infoway-inforoute.ca.

De Crescenzo, F., Economou, A., Sharpley, A. L., Gormez, A., & Quested, D. J. (2017). Actigraphic features of bipolar disorder: A systematic review and meta-analysis. *Sleep medicine reviews, 33,* 58–69. https://doi.org/10.1016/j. smrv.2016.05.003

DeRubeis, R. J., Siegle, G. J., & Hollon, S. D. (2008). Cognitive therapy versus medication for depression: treatment outcomes and neural mechanisms. *Nature reviews. Neuroscience,* 9(10), 788–796. https://doi.org/10.1038/nrn2345

Digital Around the World - DataReportal – Global Digital Insights. DataReportal. (n.d.). https://datareportal.com/global-digital-overview#:~:text=The%20number%20of%20internet%20users,900%2C000%20new%20users%20each%20

day.

ePST online problem-solving treatment for depression, a form of CBT (cognitive-behavioral therapy). EverMind. (n.d.). https://www.evermindgroup.com/epst-helps.

Government of Canada. (2021). *Impacts on Mental Health*. Government of Canada,
Statistics Canada. https://www150.statcan.gc.ca/n1/pub/11-631-x/2020004/s3-eng.htm.

Hatcher, S., Mahajan, S., Schellenberg, M., & Thapliyal, A. (2014) *E-Mental Health in Canada: Transforming the Mental Health System Using Technology*. (2014). Ottawa, ON: Mental
Health Commission of Canada. Retrieved from:http://www.mentalhealthcommission.ca.

Infoway. (n.d.). *e-Mental Health: Canada Health Infoway*. Canada Health Infoway / Inforoute
Santé Canada. https://www.infoway-inforoute.ca/en/solutions/e-mental-health.

Johnson, C., Andronis, C., Antoniadis, J., Gunn, J., Howell, C., & Orman, J. (2015). *e-Mental Health Guide*. https://www.racgp.org.au/download/Documents/Guidelines/e-Mental%20health/e-mentalhealthguide.pdf.

Lal, S. (2019). E-mental health: Promising advancements in policy, research, and practice. Healthcare Management Forum, 32(2), 56–62. https://doi.org/10.1177/0840470418818583

Marowits, R. (2020, May 15). *Internet usage has risen sharply amid coronavirus pandemic, providers say.* Global News. https://globalnews.ca/news/6946816/canadians-internet-coronavirus-providers/.

Mental Health. CMHA Ontario. (n.d.). https://ontario.cmha.ca/provincial-mental-health-supports/.

Mental Illness and Addiction: Facts and Statistics. CAMH. (n.d.). https://www.camh.ca/en/driving-change/the-crisis-is-real/mental-health-statistics.

Merry S N, Stasiak K, Shepherd M, Frampton C, Fleming T, Lucassen M F G et al. The effectiveness of SPARX, a computerised self help intervention for adolescents seeking help for depression: randomised controlled non-inferiority trial BMJ 2012; 344 :e2598 doi:10.1136/bmj.e2598

Our Story. Strongest Families Institute. (2021). https://strongestfamilies.com/our-story/.

Ryu S. (2012). Telemedicine: Opportunities and Developments in Member States: Report on the

Second Global Survey on eHealth 2009 (Global Observatory for eHealth Series, Volume 2). *Healthcare Informatics Research, 18*(2), 153–155. https://doi.org/10.4258/hir.2012.18.2.153

SPARX. sparx.org.nz. (2009). http://www.sparx.org.nz/.

Strongest Families Program. (2021) Bridge the gapp. https://nl.bridgethegapp.ca/adult/online-programs/strongest-families-program/.

Watson, A. (2021). *Daily time spent with media among adults in Canada 2020.* Statista.https://www.statista.com/statistics/237478/daily-time-spent-with-media-among-adults-in-canada/.

The Discovery of E-mental Health

About ISMHO. ISHMO. (n.d.). https://ismho.org/ismho/about-ismho/.

About Psych Central. (n.d.). https://psychcentral.com/about.

Ainsworth, M. (n.d.). Internet Therapy Guide: History and Survey of E-Therapy. https://www.metanoia.org/imhs/history.htm.

Bryant, M. (2021). *20 years ago today, the World Wide Web opened to the public.* TNW Insider. https://thenextweb.com/news/20-years-ago-today-the-world-wide-web-opened-to-the-public.

Godleski, L., Darkins, A., & Peters, J. (2012). Outcomes of 98,609 U.S. Department of Veterans
Affairs Patients Enrolled in Telemental Health Services, 2006–2010. *Psychiatric
Services, 63*(4), 383–385. https://doi.org/10.1176/appi.ps.201100206

Green, D. (n.d.). *Dr. Dror Green: The History of Online Psychotherapy*. The History of Online
Psychotherapy. http://www.psychom.com/Onlinehistory_en.html.

Hull, T. D., & Mahan, K. (2017). A Study of Asynchronous Mobile-Enabled SMS Text
Psychotherapy. *Telemedicine and e-Health, 23*(3), 240–247.
https://doi.org/10.1089/tmj.2016.0114.

Jorm, A. F., Morgan, A. J., & Malhi, G. S. (2013). The future of e-mental health. *The Australian
and New Zealand journal of psychiatry, 47*(2), 104–106.
https://doi.org/10.1177/0004867412474076.

Kessler, D., Lewis, G., Kaur, S., Wiles, N., King, M., Weich, S., … Peters, T. J. (2009).
Therapist-delivered internet psychotherapy for depression in primary care: a randomised
controlled trial. *The Lancet, 374*(9690), 628–634. https://doi.org/10.1016/s0140-6736(09)61257-5.

Lal, S., & Adair, C. E. (2014). E-mental health: a rapid

review of the literature. *Psychiatric services (Washington, D.C.), 65*(1), 24–32. https://doi. org/10.1176/appi.ps.201300009.

Lang , S., & February 20, 2007. (2007, February 20). *For two decades, Dear Uncle Ezra, world's first online advice column, has aided the perplexed, the shy and the confused.* Cornell Chronicle. https://news. cornell.edu/stories/2007/02/any-person-any-question-ask-dear-uncle-ezra-advice#:~:text=Over%20two%20 decades%20%22Dear%20Uncle,in%20more%20than%20 30%20countries.&text=The%20actual%20Uncle%20 Ezra%20is,to%2020%20questions%20a%20week.

Mayo Clinic Staff. (2020, May 15). *Managing your health in the age of Wi-Fi. Mayo Clinic.* https://www.mayoclinic.org/healthy-lifestyle/ consumer-health/in-depth/telehealth/art-200 44878.

Mental Health. CMHA Ontario. (n.d.). https://ontario. cmha.ca/about-cmha/history-of-cmha/.

Rauch, W. byJ., Rauch, J., Joseph Rauch Staff Writer at Talkspace, Su, W. byE., & Su, E. (2018). *The History of Online Therapy.* Talkspace.https:// www.talkspace.com/blog/history-online-therapy/#:~:text=In%201995%20therapist%20John%20 Grohol,of%20donating%20money%20to%20him.

Riper, H., Andersson, G., Christensen, H., Cuijpers, P., Lange, A., & Eysenbach, G. (2010). Theme issue on e-mental health: a growing field in

internet research. *Journal of medical Internet research,*
12(5), e74. https://doi.org/10.2196/jmir.1713.

Ruwaard, J., Lange, A., Schrieken, B., & Emmelkamp, P.
(2011). Efficacy and effectiveness of
online cognitive behavioral treatment: a decade of
interapy research. *Studies in health*
technology and informatics, 167, 9–14.

Wagner, B., Horn, A. B., & Maercker, A. (2014). Internet-
based versus face-to-face
cognitive-behavioral intervention for depression: A
randomized controlled non-inferiority
trial. *Journal of Affective Disorders, 152-154,* 113–121.
https://doi.org/10.1016/j.jad.2013.06.032.

Who We Are. Who We Are | Mental Health Commission
of Canada. (n.d.).
https://www.mentalhealthcommission.ca/English/
who-we-are.

Wozney, L., Newton, A. S., Gehring, N. D., Bennett, K.,
Huguet, A., Hartling, L., Dyson, M. P.,
& McGrath, P. (2017). Implementation of eMental
Health care: viewpoints from key
informants from organizations and agencies with
eHealth mandates. *BMC medical informatics and decision*
making, 17(1), 78. https://doi.org/10.1186/s12911-017-
0474-9.

Arsenault-Lapierre, G., Kim, C. & Turecki, G. Psychiatric diagnoses in 3275 suicides: a meta-analysis. *BMC Psychiatry 4*, 37 (2004). https://doi.org/10.1186/1471-244X-4-37

Brännlund, A., Strandh, M., & Nilsson, K. (2017). Mental-health and educational achievement: the link between poor mental-health and upper secondary school completion and grades. *Journal of Mental Health (Abingdon, England)*, 26(4), 318–325. https://doi.org/10.1080/09638237.2017.1294739

Epigenetics. (n.d.) In *National Human Genome Research Institute.* https://www.genome.gov/genetics-glossary/Epigenetics

Jaya S. Khushalani, Jin Qin, John Cyrus, Natasha Buchanan Lunsford, Sun Hee Rim, Xuesong Han, K. Robin Yabroff & Donatus U. Ekwueme (2018) Systematic review of healthcare costs related to mental health conditions among cancer survivors, *Expert Review of Pharmacoeconomics & Outcomes Research*, 18:5, 505-517, DOI: 10.1080/14737167.2018.1485097

Kaneita, Y., Yokoyama, E., Harano, S., Tamaki, T., Suzuki, H., Munezawa, T., … Ohida, T. (2008). Associations between sleep disturbance and

mental health status: A
longitudinal study of Japanese junior high school
students. Sleep Medicine, 10(7), 780–786. https://doi.
org/10.1016/j.sleep.2008.06.014

Kenney, S. R., DiGuiseppi, G. T., Meisel, M. K.,
Balestrieri, S. G., & Barnett, N. P.
(2018). Poor mental health, peer drinking norms, and
alcohol risk in a social
network of first-year college students. Addictive
Behaviors, 84, 151–159. https://doi.org/10.1016/j.
addbeh.2018.04.012

Mental Health (n.d.) In *Oxford Dictionary*.
https://www.lexico.com/definition/mental_health

Monaco, A.P. An epigenetic, transgenerational model of
increased mental health
disorders in children, adolescents and young adults.
Eur J Hum Genet 29,
387–395 (2021). https://doi.org/10.1038/s41431-020-
00726-4

Ohrnberger, J., Fichera, E., & Sutton, M. (2017). The
relationship between physical and
mental health: *A mediation analysis. Social Science &
Medicine* (1982), 195,
42–49. https://doi.org/10.1016/j.socscimed.2017.11.008

Olesen, S. C., Olesen, S. C., Butterworth, P.,
Butterworth, P., Rodgers, B., & Rodgers,
B. (2012). Is poor mental health a risk factor for

retirement? Findings from a
longitudinal population survey. *Social Psychiatry and Psychiatric Epidemiology, 47*(5), 735–744. https://doi.org/10.1007/s00127-011-0375-7

Staiger, T., Waldmann, T., Oexle, N., Wigand, M., & Rüsch, N. (2018). Intersections of
discrimination due to unemployment and mental health problems: the role of
double stigma for job- and help-seeking behaviors. *Social Psychiatry and Psychiatric Epidemiology, 53*(10), 1091–1098. https://doi.org/10.1007/s00127-018-1535-9

Importance of E-mental Health in Today's Society

De', R., Pandey, N., & Pal, A. (2020). Impact of digital surge during Covid-19 pandemic: A viewpoint on research and practice. *International Journal Of Information Management, 55,* 102171. https://doi.org/10.1016/j.ijinfomgt.2020.102171

Dobson, K. G., Vigod, S. N., Mustard, C., & Smith, P. M. (2020). *Health Reports Trends in the prevalence of depression and anxiety disorders among working-age Canadian adults between 2000 and 2016.* https://doi.org/10.25318/82-003-x202001200002-eng

Gadermann, A., Thomson, K., Richardson, C., Gagné, M., McAuliffe, C., Hirani, S., & Jenkins, E. (2021). Examining the impacts of the COVID-19 pandemic on family mental health in Canada: findings from a national cross-sectional study. *BMJ Open, 11*(1), e042871. https://doi.org/10.1136/bmjopen-2020-042871

Hossain, M., Tasnim, S., Sultana, A., Faizah, F., Mazumder, H., & Zou, L. et al. (2020). Epidemiology of mental health problems in COVID-19: a review. *F1000research, 9,* 636. https://doi.org/10.12688/f1000research.24457.1

Jeong, D., Cheng, M., St-Jean, M., & Jalali, A. (2019). Evaluation of eMentalHealth.ca, a Canadian Mental Health Website Portal: Mixed Methods Assessment. *JMIR Mental Health, 6*(9), e13639. https://doi.org/10.2196/13639

Monaghesh, E., & Hajizadeh, A. (2020). The role of telehealth during COVID-19 outbreak: a systematic review based on current evidence. *BMC Public Health, 20*(1). https://doi.org/10.1186/s12889-020-09301-4

Moock, J. (2014). Support from the Internet for Individuals with Mental Disorders: Advantages and Disadvantages of e-Mental Health Service Delivery. *Frontiers In Public Health, 2.* https://doi.org/10.3389/fpubh.2014.00065

Singh, S., Roy, D., Sinha, K., Parveen, S., Sharma, G., & Joshi, G. (2020). Impact of COVID-19 and lockdown on mental health of children and adolescents: A narrative review with recommendations. *Psychiatry Research, 293,* 113429. https://doi.org/10.1016/j.psychres.2020.113429

Statistics Canada. (2020). *Impacts on Mental Health.* Statistics Canada. Retrieved 8 May 2021, from https:// www150.statcan.gc.ca/n1/pub/11-631-x/2020004/s3-eng.htm.

Statistics Canada. (2021). The Daily — *Survey on COVID-19 and Mental Health, September to December 2020.* Statistics Canada. Retrieved 8 May 2021, from https://www150.statcan.gc.ca/n1/daily-quotidien/210318/dq210318a-eng.htm.

The Royal Australian College of General Practitioners,. (2015). *e-Mental health A guide for GPs.* Victoria. Retrieved from https://www.racgp.org.au/download/Documents/Guidelines/e-Mental%20health/e-mentalhealthguide.pdf

Torous, J., Jän Myrick, K., Rauseo-Ricupero, N., & Firth, J. (2020). Digital Mental Health and COVID-19: Using Technology Today to Accelerate the Curve on Access and Quality Tomorrow. *JMIR Mental Health, 7*(3), e18848. https://doi.org/10.2196/18848

What is E-mental health?

Galderisi, S., Heinz, A., Kastrup, M., Beezhold, J., & Sartorius, N. (2015). Toward a new definition of mental health. *World Psychiatry, 14*(2), 231–233. https://doi.org/10.1002/wps.20231

World Health Organization. (2004). *Promoting mental health: concepts, emerging evidence, practice (Summary*

Report).
https://www.who.int/mental_health/evidence/en/
promoting_mhh.pdf

Statistics Canada. (2020). *Survey on COVID-19 Mental
Health, September to December 2020.*
https://www150.statcan.gc.ca/n1/daily-
quotidien/210318/dq210318a-eng.htm

Hatcher, Simon., Mahajan, S., Schellenberg, M., &
Thapliyal, A. (2014). Mental health Commision Canada.
*E-Mental health in Canada: Transforming the Mental health
System Using Technology.*
https://www.mentalhealthcommission.ca/sites/
default/files/MHCC_E-Mental_Health-Briefing_
Document_ENG_0.pdf

Mucic, D., & Hilty, D. M. (2016). *E-Mental Health.*
Springer International Publishing. https://link.
springer.com/content/pdf/10.1007/978-3-319-20852-7.
pdf

Mohr, D. C., Burns, M. N., Schueller, S. M., Clarke,
G., & Klinkman, M. (2013). Behavioral Intervention
Technologies: Evidence review and recommendations
for future research in mental health. *General Hospital
Psychiatry, 35*(4), 332–338. https://doi.org/10.1016/j.
genhosppsych.2013.03.008

Cotton, R., Hyatt, J., & Patrick, M. (2013). E-mental
health: what's all the fuss about? Mental Health
Network: NHS Confederation. https://www.

nhsconfed.org/-/media/Confederation/Files/
Publications/Documents/E-mental-health.pdf

Shalaby, R., & Agyapong, V. (2020). Peer Support in Mental Health: Literature Review. *JMIR Mental Health,* 7(6). https://doi.org/10.2196/15572

CMHA National. (2019. *The Power of Peer Support.* https://cmha.ca/the-power-of-peer-support.

Ybarra, M., & Eaton, W. (2005). Internet-based mental health interventions. *Mental Health Services Research, 7,* 75-87.

Rickwood, D., Deane, F., & Wilson, C. (2007). When and how do young people seek professional help for mental health problems? *Medical Journal of Australia,* 187(1), 35-39.

Horgan, A., & Sweeney, J. (2010). Young students' use of the Internet for mental health information and support. *Journal of Psychiatric and Mental Health Nursing,* 17, 117-123

Benefits and Possible Contraindications of E-mental Health

Moock, J. (2014, May 27). Support from the internet for individuals with mental disorders: Advantages and disadvantages of e-mental health service delivery. https://www.frontiersin.org/articles/10.3389/fpubh.2014.00065/full

Reichert, A., & Jacobs, R. (2018, November). The impact of waiting time on patient outcomes: Evidence from early intervention in PSYCHOSIS services in England. https://www.ncbi.nlm.nih.gov/pmc/articles/PMC6221005/

Situmorang, D. (2020) Online/Cyber counseling services in the COVID-19 OUTBREAK: Are they really new? - *DOMINIKUS DAVID Biondi* Situmorang. https://journals.sagepub.com/doi/full/10.1177/1542305020948170

Wise J, Waugh M, Mishkind M, Ventriglio A, Thara R, Thapliyal A, Tolentino E, Shore J, Bhugra D (2016). WPA Position Statement on e-Mental Health. *World Psychiatry Association.*

The Science of E-mental Health

Abdullah, M. H. (2005, January). *What is bibliotherapy?* https://cyc-net.org/cyc-online/cycol-0105-biblio.html

Barak, A., & Grohol, J. M. (2011). Current and Future Trends in Internet-Supported Mental Health Interventions. *Journal of Technology in Human Services,* 29(3), 155–196. https://doi.org/10.1080/15228835.2011.616939

Bauer, S., & Moessner, M. (2012). Technology-enhanced monitoring in psychotherapy and e-mental health. *Journal of Mental Health, 21*(4), 355–363. https://doi.org/10.3109/09638237.2012.667886

Bäuml, J., Froböse, T., Kraemer, S., Rentrop, M., & Pitschel-Walz, G. (2006). Psychoeducation: A Basic Psychotherapeutic Intervention for Patients With Schizophrenia and Their Families. *Schizophrenia Bulletin, 32*(Suppl 1), S1–S9. https://doi.org/10.1093/schbul/sbl017

Becker, D. (2016). *E-Mental Health: Contributions, Challenges, and Research Opportunities from a Computer Science Perspective* (pp. 928–936).

Cacioppo, J. T., Amaral, D. G., Blanchard, J. J., Cameron, J. L., Carter, C. S., Crews, D., Fiske, S., Heatherton, T., Johnson, M. K., Kozak, M. J., Levenson, R. W., Lord, C., Miller, E. K., Ochsner, K., Raichle, M. E., Shea, M. T., Taylor, S. E., Young, L. J., & Quinn, K. J. (2007). Social Neuroscience: Progress and Implications for Mental Health. *Perspectives on Psychological Science: A Journal of the Association for Psychological Science, 2*(2), 99–123. https://doi.org/10.1111/j.1745-6916.2007.00032.x

Canadian Public Health Association. (2021). *A Public Health Approach to Population Mental Wellness.* https://www.cpha.ca/sites/default/files/uploads/policy/positionstatements/2021-03-population-mental-wellness-e.pdf

Daigle, P., & Rudnick, A. (2020). Shifting to Remotely Delivered Mental Health Care: Quality Improvement in the COVID-19 Pandemic. *Psychiatry International, 1*(1), 31–35. https://doi.org/10.3390/psychiatryint1010005

Donker, T., Griffiths, K. M., Cuijpers, P., & Christensen, H. (2009). Psychoeducation for depression, anxiety and psychological distress: A meta-analysis. *BMC Medicine, 7*(1), 79. https://doi.org/10.1186/1741-7015-7-79

Ekhtiari, H., Rezapour, T., Aupperle, R. L., & Paulus, M. P. (2017). Chapter 10 - Neuroscience-informed psychoeducation for addiction medicine: A neurocognitive perspective. In T. Calvey & W. M. U. Daniels (Eds.), *Progress in Brain Research* (Vol. 235, pp. 239–264). Elsevier. https://doi.org/10.1016/bs.pbr.2017.08.013

Encyclopedia of Body Image and Human Appearance. (2012). Elsevier. https://doi.org/10.1016/C2010-1-66177-9

Fenn, K., & Byrne, M. (2013). The key principles of cognitive behavioural therapy. *InnovAiT, 6*(9), 579–585. https://doi.org/10.1177/1755738012471029

Hyman, S. E. (2000). The genetics of mental illness: Implications for practice. *Bulletin of the World Health Organization, 78*(4), 455–463.

Lal, S. (2019). E-mental health: Promising advancements in policy, research, and practice. *Healthcare Management Forum, 32*(2), 56–62. https://doi.org/10.1177/0840470418818583

Lal, S., & Adair, C. E. (2014). E-Mental Health: A Rapid Review of the Literature. *Psychiatric Services, 65*(1), 24–32. https://doi.org/10.1176/appi.ps.201300009

McGinty, K. L., Saeed, S. A., Simmons, S. C., & Yildirim, Y. (2006). Telepsychiatry and e-Mental Health Services: Potential for Improving Access to Mental Health Care. *Psychiatric Quarterly, 77*(4), 335–342. https://doi.org/10.1007/s11126-006-9019-6

Mental Health Commission of Canada. (2014). *E-Mental Health in Canada: Transforming the Mental Health System Using Technology.* https://www.mentalhealthcommission.ca/sites/default/files/MHCC_E-Mental_Health-Briefing_Document_ENG_0.pdf

OHTN Rapid Response Service. (2018). *Online mental health counselling interventions.* Ontario HIV Treatment Network. https://www.ohtn.on.ca/rapid-response-online-mental-health-counselling-interventions/

Patten, S. B. (2015). Psychiatric Epidemiology: It Is About Much More Than Prevalence. *Canadian Journal of Psychiatry. Revue Canadienne de Psychiatrie, 60*(12), 529–530.

Pereira, A. (2007). What The Cognitive Neurosciences Mean To Me. *Mens Sana Monographs, 5*(1), 158–168. https://doi.org/10.4103/0973-1229.32160

Rector, N. A. (2010). *Cognitive-behavioural therapy: An information Guide.* Centre for Addiction and Mental Health. https://www.camh.ca/-/media/files/guides-and-publications/cbt-guide-en.pdf

Richardson, P. (1997). ABC of mental health: Psychological treatments. *BMJ, 315*(7110), 733–735. https://doi.org/10.1136/bmj.315.7110.733

Riggio, R. E., & Riggio, H. R. (2012). Face and Body in Motion: Nonverbal Communication. In T. Cash (Ed.), *Encyclopedia of Body Image and Human Appearance* (pp. 425–430). Academic Press. https://doi.org/10.1016/B978-0-12-384925-0.00068-7

Riper, H., Andersson, G., Christensen, H., Cuijpers, P., Lange, A., & Eysenbach, G. (2010). Theme Issue on E-Mental Health: A Growing Field in Internet Research. *Journal of Medical Internet Research, 12*(5), e1713. https://doi.org/10.2196/jmir.1713

Schmidt, U., & Wykes, T. (2012). E-mental health – a land of unlimited possibilities. *Journal of Mental Health, 21*(4), 327–331. https://doi.org/10.3109/09638237.2012.705930

Shoemaker, E. Z., & Hilty, D. M. (2016). E-Mental Health Improves Access to Care, Facilitates Early Intervention, and Provides Evidence-Based Treatments at a Distance. In D. Mucic & D. M. Hilty (Eds.), *E-Mental Health* (pp. 43–57). Springer International Publishing. https://doi.org/10.1007/978-3-319-20852-7_3

The Australian Psychological Society. (2018). *Evidence-Based Psychological Interventions in the Treatment of Mental Disorders.* https://www.psychology.org.au/getmedia/23c6a11b-2600-4e19-9a1d-6ff9c2f26fae/

Evidence-based-psych-interventions.pdf

Titov, N., Dear, B. F., Staples, L. G., Bennett-Levy, J., Klein, B., Rapee, R. M., Andersson, G., Purtell, C., Bezuidenhout, G., & Nielssen, O. B. (2017). The first 30 months of the MindSpot Clinic: Evaluation of a national e-mental health service against project objectives. *Australian & New Zealand Journal of Psychiatry, 51*(12), 1227–1239. https://doi.org/10.1177/0004867416671598

Williams, A. D., & Andrews, G. (2013). The Effectiveness of Internet Cognitive Behavioural Therapy (iCBT) for Depression in Primary Care: A Quality Assurance Study. *PLOS ONE, 8(2)*, e57447. https://doi.org/10.1371/journal.pone.0057447

Wittchen, H.-U., Härtling, S., & Hoyer, J. (2015). Psychotherapy and Mental Health as a Psychological Science Discipline. *Verhaltenstherapie, 25*(2), 98–109. https://doi.org/10.1159/000430772

Wojtalik, J. A., Eack, S. M., Smith, M. J., & Keshavan, M. S. (2018). Using Cognitive Neuroscience to Improve Mental Health Treatment: A Comprehensive Review. *Journal of the Society for Social Work and Research, 9*(2), 223–260. https://doi.org/10.1086/697566

World Health Organization. (1948). *What is the WHO definition of health?* https://www.who.int/about/who-we-are/frequently-asked-questions

Al-Asadi, A. M., Klein, B., & Meyer, D. (2014). Posttreatment attrition and its predictors, attrition bias, and treatment efficacy of the anxiety online programs. *Journal of medical Internet research, 16*(10), e232. https://doi.org/10.2196/jmir.3513

Andersson, G., & Hedman, E. (2013). Effectiveness of Guided Internet-Based Cognitive Behavior Therapy in Regular Clinical Settings. *Verhaltenstherapie, 23*(3), 140-148. doi: 10.1159/000354779

Andersson, G., & Titov, N. (2014). Advantages and limitations of Internet-based interventions for common mental disorders. World psychiatry : official journal of the *World Psychiatric Association (WPA), 13*(1), 4–11. https://doi.org/10.1002/wps.20083

APA. (2021). APA App Advisor. Retrieved 6 May 2021, from https://www.psychiatry.org/psychiatrists/practice/mental-health-apps

Association of Canadian Psychology Regulatory Organizations (ACPRO). (2011). *Model Standards for Telepsychology Service Delivery* [Ebook]. Toronto: Association of Canadian Psychology Regulatory Organizations. Retrieved from https://acpro-aocrp.ca/wp-content/

uploads/2020/03/ACPRO-Model-Standards-for-Telepsychology-Service-Delivery.pdf

 CAMH. (2021). Apps for Mental Health. Retrieved 3 May 2021, from https://www.camh.ca/en/health-info/mental-health-and-covid-19/information-for-professionals/apps-for-mental-health

Chakrabarti S. (2015). Usefulness of telepsychiatry: A critical evaluation
of videoconferencing-based approaches. *World journal of psychiatry, 5*(3), 286–304. https://doi.org/10.5498/wjp.v5.i3.286

Chandrashekar P. (2018). Do mental health mobile apps work: evidence and recommendations
for designing high-efficacy mental health mobile apps. mHealth, 4, 6. https://doi.org/10.21037/mhealth.2018.03.02

Ćosić, K., Popović, S., Šarlija, M., Kesedžić, I., & Jovanovic, T. (2020). Artificial intelligence in prediction of mental health disorders induced by the COVID-19 pandemic among health
care workers. *Croatian medical journal, 61(3)*, 279–288. https://doi.org/10.3325/cmj.2020.61.279

D'Alfonso, S. (2020). AI in mental health. *Current Opinion In Psychology, 36*, 112-117. doi: 10.1016/j.copsyc.2020.04.005

E-Mental Health in Canada: Transforming the Mental Health System Using Technology - A Briefing Document. (2014). Mental Health Commission of Canada.

Ebert, D., Harrer, M., Apolinário-Hagen, J., & Baumeister, H. (2019). Digital Interventions for Mental Disorders: Key Features, Efficacy, and Potential for Artificial Intelligence Applications. Frontiers in Psychiatry, 583–627. https://doi.org/10.1007/978-981-32- 9721-0_29

eMentalHealth.ca. (2021). *About Us : eMentalHealth.ca.* eMentalHealth.ca Resource Directory. Retrieved 3 May 2021, from https://www.ementalhealth.ca/index. php?m=staticPage&ID=14424.

Gaebel, W. (2017). E-Mental health for mental disorders–focus on psychotic disorders and PTSD. *European Psychiatry, 41*(S1), S42–S42. https://doi.org/10.1016/j.eurpsy.2017.01.189

Geirhos, A., Lunkenheimer, F., Holl, R. W., Minden, K., Schmitt, A., Temming, S., Baumeister, H., & Domhardt, M. (2021). Involving patients' perspective in the development of an internet- and mobile-based CBT intervention for adolescents with chronic medical conditions: Findings from a qualitative study. *Internet interventions, 24,* 100383. https://doi. org/10.1016/j.invent.2021.100383

Hailey, D., Roine, R., & Ohinmaa, A. (2008). The effectiveness
of telemental health applications: a review.
Canadian journal of psychiatry. Revue canadienne de psychiatrie, 53(11), 769–778. https://doi.org/10.1177/070674370805301109

Harris B, Birnbaum R. Ethical and legal implications on the use of technology in
counselling. *Clin Soc Work J* (2015) 43(2):133–41. doi: 10.1007/s10615-014-0515-0
https://doi.org/10.2196/14897

Hubley, S., Lynch, S. B., Schneck, C., Thomas, M., & Shore, J. (2016). Review of
key telepsychiatry outcomes. *World journal of psychiatry, 6*(2), 269–282. https://doi.org/10.5498/wjp.v6.i2.269

Jeong, D., Cheng, M., St-Jean, M., & Jalali, A. (2019). Evaluation of eMentalHealth.ca,
a Canadian Mental Health Website Portal: Mixed Methods Assessment. *JMIR mental health, 6*(9), e13639. https://doi.org/10.2196/13639

JMIR. (2021). JMIR - *Journal of Medical Internet Research Themes*. Retrieved 4 May 2021,
from https://www.jmir.org/themes

Karasouli, E., & Adams, A. (2014). Assessing the Evidence for e-Resources for
Mental Health Self-Management: A Systematic Literature Review. *JMIR Mental*

Health, 1(1), e3–e3. https://doi.org/10.2196/mental.3708

Mayer, G., Gronewold, N., Alvarez, S., Bruns, B., Hilbel, T., & Schultz, J. H.
(2019). Acceptance and Expectations of Medical Experts, Students, and Patients
Toward Electronic Mental Health Apps: Cross-Sectional Quantitative and Qualitative Survey Study. *JMIR mental health, 6*(11), e14018. https://doi.org/10.2196/14018

Mental Health Commission of Canada. (2020). 9th Annual E-Mental Health
Conference Caring in a Digital World: Introducing Disruptive Change to Mental Health Care: Summary Report [Ebook]. Mental Health Commission of Canada. Retrieved from https://www.mentalhealthcommission.ca/sites/default/files/2020-09/EMental_Health_Conference_2020_Summary_Report_eng.pdf

MHCC. (2021). *Advancing the Evolution - Insights Into the State of e-Mental Health Services in Canada* | Mental Health Commission of Canada.
Mentalhealthcommission.ca. Retrieved 3 May 2021, from https://www.mentalhealthcommission.ca/English/media/3930.

Miralles, I., Granell, C., Díaz-Sanahuja, L., Van Woensel, W., Bretón-López, J., Mira,
A., Castilla, D., & Casteleyn, S. (2020). Smartphone Apps for the Treatment of

Mental Disorders: Systematic Review. *JMIR mHealth and uHealth*, 8(4), e14897.

Mucic, D., & Hilty, D. (2016). e-Mental Health (1st ed. 2016.). Springer
International Publishing. https://doi.org/10.1007/978-3-319-20852-7

Ruwaard, J., Lange, A., Schrieken, B., Dolan, C. V., & Emmelkamp, P. (2012). The effectiveness
of online cognitive behavioral treatment in routine clinical practice. *PloS one, 7*(7),
e40089. https://doi.org/10.1371/journal.pone.0040089

Schlegl, S., Bürger, C., Schmidt, L., Herbst, N., & Voderholzer, U. (2015). The potential
of technology-based psychological interventions for anorexia and bulimia nervosa: a systematic review and recommendations for future research. *Journal of medical Internet research, 17*(3), e85. https://doi.org/10.2196/jmir.3554

Schmidt, M., Fisher, A. P., Sensenbaugh, J., Ling, B., Rietta, C., Babcock, L., Kurowski, B.
G., & Wade, S. L. (2020). User experience (re)design and evaluation of a self-guided, mobile health app for adolescents with mild Traumatic Brain Injury. *Journal of formative design in learning, 4*(2), 51–64. https://doi.org/10.1007/s41686-019-00038-x

Simms, D., Gibson, K., & O'Donnell, S. (2011). To Use or Not to Use: Clinicians'

Perceptions of Telemental Health. *Canadian Psychology = Psychologie Canadienne,*
52(1), 41–51. https://doi.org/10.1037/a0022275

Stjerneklar, S., Hougaard, E., McLellan, L. F., & Thastum, M. (2019). A randomized controlled trial examining the efficacy of an internet-based cognitive behavioral therapy program for adolescents with anxiety disorders. *PloS one, 14*(9), e0222485.
https://doi.org/10.1371/journal.pone.0222485

Stoll, J., Müller, J. A., & Trachsel, M. (2020). Ethical Issues in Online Psychotherapy: A Narrative Review. *Frontiers in psychiatry, 10,* 993. https://doi.org/10.3389/fpsyt.2019.00993

Talkspace. (2021). Talkspace - #1 Rated Online Therapy, 1 Million+ Users. Talkspace.com. Retrieved 4 May 2021, from https://www.talkspace.com/#how.

Titov, N., Dear, B., Nielssen, O., Staples, L., Hadjistavropoulos, H., Nugent, M., Adlam, K., Nordgreen, T., Bruvik, K., Hovland, A., Repål, A., Mathiasen, K., Kraepelien, M., Blom, K., Svanborg, C., Lindefors, N., & Kaldo, V. (2018). ICBT in routine care: A descriptive analysis of successful clinics in five countries. *Internet Interventions : the Application of Information Technology in Mental and Behavioural Health, 13,* 108–115. https://doi.org/10.1016/j.invent.2018.07.006

Tremain, H., McEnery, C., Fletcher, K., & Murray, G. (2020). The Therapeutic Alliance in Digital Mental Health Interventions for Serious Mental Illnesses: Narrative Review. *JMIR mental health, 7*(8), e17204. https://doi.org/10.2196/17204

Wade, V. A., Eliott, J. A., & Hiller, J. E. (2014). Clinician acceptance is the key factor for sustainable telehealth services. *Qualitative health research, 24*(5), 682–694. https://doi.org/10.1177/1049732314528809

Zelmer, J., van Hoof, K., Notarianni, M., van Mierlo, T., Schellenberg, M., & Tannenbaum, C. (2018). An Assessment Framework for e-Mental Health Apps in Canada: Results of a Modified Delphi Process. *JMIR mHealth and uHealth, 6*(7), e10016–e10016. https://doi.org/10.2196/10016

E-mental Health: A Safe Environment for Everyone

Al-Alawi, M., McCall, R. K., Sultan, A., Al Balushi, N., Al-Mahrouqi, T., Al Ghailani, A., Al Sabti, H., Al-Maniri, A., Panchatcharam, S. M., & Al Sinawi, H. (2021). Efficacy of a Six-Week-Long Therapist-Guided Online Therapy Versus Self-help Internet-Based Therapy for COVID-19–Induced Anxiety and Depression: Open-label, Pragmatic, Randomized Controlled Trial. *JMIR Mental Health, 8*(2). https://doi.org/10.2196/26683

Alvarez-Jimenez, M., Rice, S., D'Alfonso, S., Leicester, S., Bendall, S., Pryor, I., Russon, P., McEnery, C., Santesteban-Echarri, O., Da Costa, G., Gilbertson, T., Valentine, L., Solves, L., Ratheesh, A., McGorry, P. D., & Gleeson, J. (2020). A Novel Multimodal Digital Service (Moderated Online Social Therapy+) for Help-Seeking Young People Experiencing Mental Ill-Health: Pilot Evaluation Within a National Youth E-Mental Health Service. *Journal of Medical Internet Research, 22*(8). https://doi.org/10.2196/17155

Andersson, G., & Titov, N. (2014). Advantages and limitations of Internet-based interventions for common mental disorders. *World Psychiatry, 13(1)*, 4–11. https://doi.org/10.1002/wps.20083

Apps for Mental Health. (2018). CAMH. https://www.camh.ca/en/health-info/mental-health-and-covid-19/information-for-professionals/apps-for-mental-health

Balconi, M., Fronda, G., Venturella, I., & Crivelli, D. (2017). Conscious, pre-conscious and unconscious mechanisms in emotional behaviour. Some applications to the mindfulness approach with wearable devices. *Applied Sciences, 7,* 1–14. https://doi.org/10.3390/app7121280

Batterham P, Sunderland M, Calear A, Christensen H, Teesson M, Kay-Lambkin F. (2015). Case for Action proposal: Translation of e-mental health services for depression. *National Health and Medical Research Council, 1,* 21

Baumel A, Muench F, Edan S, Kane JM. (2019). Objective user engagement with mental health apps: systematic search and panel-based usage analysis. *J Med Internet Res, 21*(9), e14567

Berger T. (2017). The therapeutic alliance in internet interventions: a narrative review and suggestions for future research. *Psychother Res., 27*(5), 511–524. doi:10.10 80/10503307.2015.1119908

Clement, S., Brohan, E., Jeffery, D., Henderson, C., Hatch, S. L., & Thornicroft, G. (2012). Development and psychometric properties the Barriers to Access to Care Evaluation scale (BACE) related to people with mental ill health. *BMC Psychiatry, 12*(1), 36. https://doi.org/10.1186/1471-244X-12-36

Clement, S., Schauman, O., Graham, T., Maggioni, F., Evans-Lacko, S., Bezborodovs, N., ... Thornicroft, G. (2015). What is the impact of mental health-related stigma on help-seeking? A systematic review of quantitative and qualitative studies. *Psychological Medicine, 45*(1), 11–27. https://doi.org/10.1017/S0033291714000129

Ho CS, Chee CY, Ho RC. (2020). Mental health strategies to combat the psychological impact of COVID-19 beyond paranoia and panic. *Ann Acad Med Singap., 49*(3), 155–160.

Hunkin, H., King, D. L., & Zajac, I. T. (2020). Perceived acceptability of wearable devices for the treatment of mental health problems. *Journal of Clinical Psychology*, *76*(6), 987–1003. https://doi.org/10.1002/jclp.22934

Karyotaki E, Ebert DD, Donkin L, Riper H, Twisk J, Burger S, Rozental A, Lange A, Williams AD, Zarski AC, Geraedts A, van Straten A, Kleiboer A, Meyer B, Ünlü Ince BB, Buntrock C, Lehr D, Snoek FJ, Andrews G, Andersson G, Choi I, Ruwaard J, Klein JP, Newby JM, Schröder J, Laferton JAC, Van Bastelaar K, Imamura K, Vernmark K, Boß L, Sheeber LB, Kivi M, Berking M, Titov N, Carlbring P, Johansson R, Kenter R, Perini S, Moritz S, Nobis S, Berger T, Kaldo V, Forsell Y, Lindefors N, Kraepelien M, Björkelund C, Kawakami N, Cuijpers P. (2018). Do guided internet-based interventions result in clinically relevant changes for patients with depression? An individual participant data meta-analysis. *Clin Psychol Rev.*, *63*, 80–92. doi:10.1016/j.cpr.2018.06.007.

Lederman R, Wadley G, Gleeson J, Bendall S, Álvarez-Jiménez M. (2014). Moderated online social therapy. *ACM Trans Comput-Hum Interact*, *21*(1), 1-26

Luoma, J. B., Kohlenberg, B. S., Hayes, S. C., Bunting, K., & Rye, A. K. (2008). Reducing self-stigma in substance abuse through acceptance and commitment therapy: Model, manual development, and pilot outcomes. *Addiction Research & Theory*, *16*(2), 149–165. https://doi.org/10.1080/16066350701850295

Meurk, C., Leung, J., Hall, W., Head, B. W., & Whiteford, H. (2016). Establishing and Governing e-Mental Health Care in Australia: A Systematic Review of Challenges and A Call For Policy-Focussed Research. *Journal of Medical Internet Research, 18*(1). https://doi.org/10.2196/jmir.4827

Mohr DC, Weingardt KR, Reddy M, Schueller SM. (2017). Three problems with current digital mental health research . . . and three things we can do about them. *Psychiatr Serv, 68*(5), 427-429

Nicholas, J., Huckvale, K., Larsen, M. E., Basu, A., Batterham, P. J., Shaw, F., & Sendi, S. (2017). Issues for eHealth in psychiatry: Results of an expert survey. *Journal of Medical Internet Research, 19*(2), e55. https://doi.org/10.2196/jmir. 6957

Richards D, Viganó N. (2013). Online counseling: a narrative and critical review of the literature. *J Clin Psychol, 69*(9), 994-1011

Salaheddin K, Mason B. (2016). Identifying barriers to mental health help-seeking among young adults in the UK: a cross-sectional survey. *Br J Gen Pract, 66*(651), e686-e692

Saxena S, Funk MK, Chisholm D. (2015). Comprehensive mental health action plan 2013-2020. *East Mediterr Health J, 21*(7), 461-463

Veterans Affairs Canada. (2019). *PTSD Coach Canada - Mobile Applications - Stay Connected - Veterans Affairs Canada.* Veterans.gc.ca. https://www.veterans.gc.ca/

eng/resources/stay-connected/mobile-app/ptsd-coach-canada

Wallin, E., Maathz, P., Parling, T., & Hursti, T. (2018). Self-stigma and the intention to seek psychological help online compared to face-to-face. *Journal of Clinical Psychology, 74*(7), 1207–1218. https://doi.org/10.1002/jclp.22583

Weisel KK, Fuhrmann LM, Berking M, Baumeister H, Cuijpers P, Ebert DD. (2019). Standalone smartphone apps for mental health-a systematic review and meta-analysis. *NPJ Digit Med, 2,* 118

Wind TR, Rijkeboer M, Andersson G, Riper H. (2020). The COVID-19 pandemic: The 'black swan' for mental health care and a turning point for e-health. *Internet Interv., 20,* 100317. doi:10.1016/j.invent.2020.100317.

Ethics, Confidentiality, and Legal Issues

Alexander Rozental, Johanna Boettcher, Gerhard Andersson, Brad Schmidt & Per Carlbring (2015) Negative Effects of Internet Interventions: A Qualitative Content Analysis of Patients' Experiences with Treatments Delivered Online, Cognitive Behaviour Therapy, 44:3, 223-236, DOI: 10.1080/16506073.2015.1008033

Alleman, J. (2002). Online counseling: The Internet and mental health treatment. Psychotherapy: Theory, Research, Practice, Training, 39(2), 199-209.

Berk M, Parker G. The elephant on the couch: side-effects of psychotherapy. Aust NZ J Psychiatry. 2009;43(9):787–94.

Boddy, J., & Dominelli, L. (2017). Social media and social work: The challenges of a new ethical space. *Australian Social Work, 70*(2), 172–184. doi:10.1080/03124 07X.2016.1224907

Borcsa, M., & Pomini, V. (2017). Virtual relationships and systemic practices in the digital era. *Contemporary Family Therapy, 39*(4), 239–248. doi:10.1007/s10591-017-9446-6

Canadian Psychological Association. (2017). Canadian code of ethics for psychologists. Fourth edition. Ottawa, ON: Author. Retrieve from https://cpa.ca/docs/File/Ethics/CPA_Code_2017_4thEd.pdf

Cheng, Q. F., Chang, S. F., & Yip, P. S. F.(2012). Opportunities and challenges of online data collection for suicide prevention. *Lancet, 26*(379), 53–54. doi:10.1016/S0140-6736(12)60856-3

Childress, C. A. (2000). Ethical issues in providing online psychotherapeutic interventions. *JMIR, 2*(1), E5–E5. doi:10.2196/jmir.2.1.e5

Christensen, H., Griffiths, K. M., & Evans, K.(2002). E-mental health in Australia: Implications of the internet and related technologies for policy (Information Strategy Committee Discussion Paper no.

3). ACT, Australia: Centre for Mental Health Research, Australian National University.

Cosgrove, V., Gliddon, E., Berk, L. et al. Online ethics: where will the interface of mental health and the internet lead us?. *Int J Bipolar Disord 5, 26* (2017). https://doi.org/10.1186/s40345-017-0095-3

Coviello, L., Sohn, Y., Kramer, A. D. I.,Marlow, C., Franceschetti, M., Christakis, N.A., & Fowler, J. H. (2014). Detectingemotional contagion in massive socialnetworks. *PloS One, 9*(3), e90315.doi:10.1371/journal.pone.0090315

Disclosure of Suicidal Thoughts during an e-Mental Health Intervention: Relational Ethics Meets Actor-Network Theory. www.tandfonline.com/doi/full/10.1080/10508422.2019.1691003?casa_token=253ciL1a6x8AAAAA%3AJyChov73By-hI6z1CVqls-spYvKZHk2-rx0umgPUIw6N7cL42h7Dl0ngS885C-EDfj6AEiMLpbQW5Q

Dunlop, S., More, E., & Romer, D. (2011).Where do youth learn about suicides onthe internet, and what influence does thishave on suicidal ideation? *Journal of ChildPsychology and Psychiatry, 52,* 1073–1080. doi:10.1111/j.1469-7610.2011.02416.x

Ellison, N. B., Steinfield, C., & Lampe, C.(2007). The benefits of facebook 'friends': Social capital and college students' use of online social network sites. *Journal of Computer-Mediated Communication, 12*(4), 1143–1168.

doi:10.1111/j.1083-6101.2007.00367.x

Faurholt-Jepsen M, Frost M, Ritz C, Christensen EM, Jacoby AS, Mikkelsen RL, et al. Daily electronic self-monitoring in bipolar disorder using smartphones—the MONARCA I trial: a randomized, placebo-controlled, single-blind, parallel group trial. *Psychol Med.* *2015;*45(13):2691–704.

Feijt, M. A., de Kort, Y. A. W., Bongers, I. M. B., & Ijsselsteijn, W. A. (2018). Perceived drivers and barriers to the adoption of emental health by psychologists: The construction of the levels of adoption of emental health model. *Journal of Medical Internet Research, 20*(4), e153. doi:10.2196/jmir.9485

Frankel , S. A. (2000). Watch out for the "Third Man Death." Retrieved June 22, 2006, from http://www.psychboard.ca.gov/pubs/12_2000.pdf.

Granovetter, M. (1983). The strength of weak ties: A network theory revisited. *Sociological Theory, 1,* 201–233. doi:10.2307/202051

Guidelines for the practice of telepsychology. (n.d.). Retrieved from https://www.apa.org/practice/guidelines/telepsychology

Heron, K., & J.M., S. (2010). Ecological Momentary Interventions: Incorporating Mobile Technology Into Psychosocial and Health Behavior Treatments. British Journal of Health Psychology, 15(1), 1-39.

205

Humphreys, K., Winzelberg, A., & Klaw, E. (2000). Psychologists' ethical responsibilities in Internet-based groups: Issues, strategies and a call for dialogue. Professional Psychology: Research and Practice, 39(2), 493-496.

Kay-Lambkin, F. J., Baker, A. L., Geddes, J., Hunt, S. A., Woodcock, K. L., Teesson, M., … Thornton, L. (2015). The iTreAD project: A study protocol for a randomised controlled clinical trial of online treatment and social networking for binge drinking and depression in young people. BMC Public Health, 15, 1025. doi:10.1186/s12889-015-2365-2

Kramer, A. D. I., Guillory, J. E., & Hancock, J.T. (2014). Experimental evidence ofmassive-scale emotional contagionthrough social networks. Proceedings ofthe National Academy of Sciences, 111(24),8788. doi:10.1073/pnas.1320040111

Lal, S., & Adair, C. E. (2014). E-mental health: A rapid review of the literature. Psychiatric Services, 65(1), 24–32. doi:10.1176/appi.ps.201300009

Lannin, D., & Scott, N. (2013). Social networking ethics: Developing best practices for the new small world. Professional Psychology: Research and Practice, 44, 135–141. doi:10.1037/a0031794

Lehavot, K., Ben-Zeev, D., & Neville, R. E.(2012). Ethical considerations and social media: A case of suicidal postings on facebook. Journal of Dual Diagnosis, 8(4),

341–346. doi:10.1080/15504263.2012.718928

Manhaul-Baugus , M. (2001). Etherapy: Practical, ethical, and legal issues . *Cyberpsychology and Behavior* , 4 (5), 551– 563 .

Mental Health Commission of Canada. (2014.). *E-Mental Health in Canada: Transforming the Mental Health System Using Technology.*

Notredame, C., Grandgenevre, P., Pauwels, N., Morgiève, M., Wathelet, M., Vaiva, G., & Séguin, M. (2018). Leveraging the web and social media to promote access to care among suicidal individuals. *Frontiers in Psychology, 9*, 1338. doi:10.3389/fpsyg.2018.01338

Novotney, A. (2017). A growing wave of online therapy. *Monitor on Psychology, 48(2)*, 48. Retrieved from https://www.apa.org/monitor/2017/02/online-therapy

Prensky, M. (2001). Digital natives, digital immigrants part 1. *On the Horizon, 9(5)*, 1–6. doi:10.1108/10748120110424816

Reamer, F. G. (2013). Boundary issues in social work: Managing dual relationships. In D. A. Sisti, A. L. Caplan, & H. Rimon-Greenspan, *Applied ethics in mental health care: An interdisciplinary reader*(pp. 329–349). Cambridge, MA: MIT Press.

Reynolds, D. J., Stiles, W. B., Bailer, A. J., & Hughes, M. R. (2013). Impact of exchanges and client–therapist alliance in online-text psychotherapy. *Cyberpsychology,*

Behavior, and Social Networking, 16(5), 370-377. doi: 10.1089/cyber.2012.0195

Riccio, J. R. (2013). *All The Web's a Stage: The Dramaturgy of Young Adult Social Media Use* (Master of Arts). Syracuse University, Syracuse, NY.

Rice, S., Robinson, J., Bendall, S., Hetrick, S., Cox, G., Bailey, E., ... Alvarez-Jimenez, M.(2016). Online and social media suicide prevention interventions for young people: A focus on implementation and moderation. *Journal of the Canadian Academy of Child and Adolescent Psychiatry, 25*(2), 80–86.

Robinson, J., Rodrigues, M., Fisher, S., Bailey, E., & Herrman, H. (2015). Social media and suicide prevention: Findings from a stakeholder survey. *Shanghai Archives of Psychiatry, 27*(1), 27–35. doi:10.11919/j.issn.1002-0829.214133

Rosik , C. H. , & Brown , R. (2001). Professional use of the Internet: Legal and ethical issues in a member care environment . *Journal of Psychology and Theology , 2* , 106 – 120 .

Seabrook, E. M., Kern, M. L., & Rickard, N.S. (2016). Social networking sites,depression, and anxiety: A systematicreview. *JMIR Mental Health, 3*(4), e50. doi:10.2196/mental.5842

Shalini, L., & Carol, E. A. (2014). E-mental health: A rapid review of the literature. *Psychiatric Services, 65*(1),

24–32. doi:10.1176/appi.ps.201300009

Sharkey, S., Jones, R., Smithson, J., Hewis, E., Emmens, T., Ford, T., & Owens, C.(2011). Ethical practice in internet research involving vulnerable people: Lessons from a self-harm discussion forum study (SharpTalk). *Journal of Medical Ethics, 37*(12), 752–758. doi:10.1136/medethics-2011-100080

Simon, C., & Mosavel, M. (2011). Getting personal: Ethics and identity in global health research. *Developing World Bioethics, 11*(2), 82–92. doi:10.1111/j.1471-8847.2011.00297.x

Stern, S. R. (2003). Encountering distressing information in online research: A consideration of legal and ethical responsibilities. *New Media & Society, 5*(2), 249–266. doi:10.1177/1461444803005002006

Stofle , G. S. (1996). Thoughts about online psychotherapy: Ethical and practical considerations. Retrieved June 21, 2006, from http://www.members.aol.com/stofle/index.htm

Team, GoodTherapy Editor. "Are There Any Limitations to Online Therapy." GoodTherapy. GoodTherapy, 07 Oct. 2019. Web. 08 May 2021.

The Royal Australian and New Zealand College of Psychiatrists. (2019). *Benefits of e-mental health treatments and interventions.* Retrieved from https://www.ranzcp.org/news-policy/policy-and-advocacy/positionstatements/benefits-of-e-mentalhealth-treatments-and-interve

Wagner, B., Horn, A. B., & Maercker, A. (2014). Internet-based versus face-to-face cognitive-behavioral intervention for depression: A randomized controlled non-inferiority trial. *Journal of Affective Disorders, 152-154*, 113-121. Retrieved from https://www.sciencedirect.com/science/article/abs/pii/S0165032713005120?via%3Dihub

Webb, S. (2001). Avatarculture: Narrative, power and identity in virtual world environments. *Information, Communication & Society, 4*(4), 560–594. doi:10.1080/13691180110097012

White, A., Kavanagh, D., Stallman, H., Klein, B., Kay-Lambkin, F., Proudfoot, J., … Young, R. (2010). Online alcohol interventions: A systematic review. *JMIR, 12*(5), e62. doi:10.2196/jmir.1479

Detractors and Critics of E-mental Health

Apolinário-Hagen, J., Fritsche, L., Bierhals, C., & Salewski, C. (2018). Improving attitudes toward e-mental health services in the general population via psychoeducational information material: A randomized controlled trial. *Internet Interventions, 12*, 141–149. https://doi.org/10.1016/j.invent.2017.12.002

Apolinário-Hagen, J., Kemper, J., & Stürmer, C. (2017). Public Acceptability of E-Mental Health Treatment

Services for Psychological Problems: A Scoping Review. *JMIR Mental Health, 4*(2). https://doi.org/10.2196/mental.6186

Eysenbach, G. (2005). The Law of Attrition. *Journal of Medical Internet Research, 7*(1), e402. https://doi.org/10.2196/jmir.7.1.e11

Hoy, T., & Lee, R. (2021, May 1). *How Much Does An Online Counselling Chat Cost? How To Find The Best Online Therapy In 2021 | BetterHelp.* https://www.betterhelp.com/advice/chat/how-much-does-an-online-counseling-chat-cost/

Lorenz, T. (2018, October 12). *YouTube Stars Are Being Accused of Profiting Off Fans' Depression.* The Atlantic. https://www.theatlantic.com/technology/archive/2018/10/youtube-stars-accused-of-profiting-off-depression-betterhelp-shane-dawson-phillip-defranco-elle-mills/572803/

Marshall, J. M., Dunstan, D. A., & Bartik, W. (2020). Clinical or gimmickal: The use and effectiveness of mobile mental health apps for treating anxiety and depression. *Australian & New Zealand Journal of Psychiatry, 54*(1), 20–28. https://doi.org/10.1177/0004867419876700

Moock, J. (2014). Support from the Internet for Individuals with Mental Disorders: Advantages and Disadvantages of e-Mental Health Service Delivery. *Frontiers in Public Health, 2.* https://doi.org/10.3389/

fpubh.2014.00065

Musiat, P., Goldstone, P., & Tarrier, N. (2014). Understanding the acceptability of e-mental health — Attitudes and expectations towards computerised self-help treatments for mental health problems | *BMC Psychiatry* | Full Text. 14(109). https://bmcpsychiatry.biomedcentral.com/articles/10.1186/1471-244X-14-109

Reyes, A. T., Constantino, R. E., Arenas, R. A., Bombard, J. N., & Acupan, A. R. (2018). Exploring Challenges in Conducting E-Mental Health Research Among Asian American Women. *Asian/Pacific Island Nursing Journal, 3*(4), 139–153. https://doi.org/10.31372/20180304.1016

Stoll, J., Müller, J. A., & Trachsel, M. (2020, February 11). *Frontiers | Ethical Issues in Online Psychotherapy: A Narrative Review | Psychiatry.* https://www.frontiersin.org/articles/10.3389/fpsyt.2019.00993/full

Talkspace. (2021, April 28). *How much does Talkspace cost? – Talkspace – FAQs.* https://help.talkspace.com/hc/en-us/articles/360041531131-How-much-does-Talkspace-cost-

Wiederhold, B. K. (2020). Connecting Through Technology During the Coronavirus Disease 2019 Pandemic: Avoiding "Zoom Fatigue." *Cyberpsychology, Behavior, and Social Networking, 23*(7), 437–438. https://doi.org/10.1089/cyber.2020.29188.bkw

Williams, A., Fossey, E., Farhall, J., Foley, F., & Thomas, N. (2018). Going Online Together: The Potential for Mental Health Workers to Integrate Recovery Oriented E-Mental Health Resources Into Their Practice. *Psychiatry, 81*(2), 116–129. https://doi.org/10.1080/0033 2747.2018.1492852

How Different Cultures View E-mental Health

Aggarwal, N. (2012). Applying mobile technologies to mental health service delivery in South Asia. *Asian Journal of Psychiatry, 3*(5), 225-230 https://www.sciencedirect.com/science/article/pii/S187620181100164X?via%3Dihub

Blumenfield, S. (2020). Digital tools are REVOLUTIONIZING mental health care in the U.S. https://hbr.org/2020/12/digital-tools-are-revolutionizing-mental-health-care-in-the-u-s

Karasz, A., Gany, F., Escobar, J., Flores, C., Prasad, L., Inman, A., Kalasapudi, V., Kosi, R., Murthy, M., Leng, J., & Diwan, S. (2019). Mental Health and Stress Among South Asians. *Journal of immigrant and minority health, 21*(1), 7–14. https://doi.org/10.1007/s10903-016-0501-4

Mucic, D., Hilty, D. M., & Yellowlees, P. M. (2016). E-Mental health toward cross-cultural populations worldwide. *E-Mental Health 77*-91. doi:10.1007/978-3-319-20852-7_5

Satcher, D. (2001). Office of the Surgeon General. *Chapter 2 culture counts: The influence of culture and society on mental health*. https://www.ncbi.nlm.nih.gov/books/NBK44249/

Spanhel, K., Balci, S., Baumeister, H., Bengel, J., & Sander, L. (2020). Systemic Reviews. *Cultural adaptation of internet- and mobile-based interventions for mental disorders: A systematic review protocol, 207(9)* https://systematicreviewsjournal.biomedcentral.com/articles/10.1186/s13643-020-01438-y

Future Technologies for E-mental Health

Abilify MyCite. (n.d.). *How the ABILIFY MYCITE® System works*. How the ABILIFY MYCITE® System Works - ABILIFY MYCITE® System. https://www.abilifymycite.com/how-mycite-works.

Benedek, M., & Kaernbach, C. (2010). A continuous measure of phasic electrodermal activity. *Journal of Neuroscience Methods, 190*(1), 80–91. https://doi.org/10.1016/j.jneumeth.2010.04.028

Critchley, H., & Nagai, Y. (2020). Electrodermal Activity (EDA). *Encyclopedia of Behavioral Medicine, 741–744.* https://doi.org/10.1007/978-3-030-39903-0_13

Debard, G., De Witte, N., Sels, R., Mertens, M., Van Daele, T., & Bonroy, B. (2020). Making Wearable Technology Available for Mental Healthcare through an Online Platform with Stress Detection Algorithms: The

Carewear Project. *Journal of Sensors,* 2020, 1–15. https://doi.org/10.1155/2020/8846077

Grainger, C., & Barnes, R. (2021, January 5). *Digital technology & youth mental health - Part 4: What might the future look like?* WeAreAugust. https://www.weareaugust.ca/blog/digital-technology-youth-mental-health-part-4-what-might-the-future-look-like/.

Gusinsky, A. (2019, February 22). *How much does Psychotherapy Cost in Canada?* Alexandra Gusinsky Psychotherapy. https://www.mypsychotherapist.ca/how-much-does-psychotherapy-cost-in-canada/.

Humi Team. (2020). *Humi Blog.* RSS. https://www.humi.ca/blog-post/virtual-health-resources-for-canadians-during-covid-19?visitor_id=x8yXPHF9OBdntO.

Jones, D. (2018, May 10). *The Blood Volume Pulse - Biofeedback Basics.* Anatomical Concepts. https://www.biofeedback-tech.com/articles/2016/3/24/the-blood-volume-pulse-biofeedback-basics#:~:text=The%20blood%20volume%20pulse%20.

Jorm, A. F., Morgan, A. J., & Malhi, G. S. (2013). The future of e-mental health. Australian & New Zealand *Journal of Psychiatry.* https://novascotia.cmha.ca/wp-content/uploads/2017/06/The-future-of-e-mental-health.pdf.

Knable, M. (2020, August 31). *Muse Technology Professional Review.* One Mind PsyberGuide. https://onemindpsyberguide.org/expert-review/muse-professional-review/.

Maples-Keller, J. L., Bunnell, B. E., Kim, S.-J., & Rothbaum, B. O. (2017). The Use of Virtual Reality Technology in the Treatment of Anxiety and Other Psychiatric Disorders. *Harvard Review of Psychiatry, 25*(3), 103–113. https://doi.org/10.1097/hrp.0000000000000138

Marill, M. C. (2020). *How a Vibrating Smartwatch Could Be Used to Stop Nightmares.* Wired. https://www.wired.com/story/how-a-vibrating-smartwatch-could-be-used-to-stop-nightmares/.

Martin, S. (2019, June 24). *Virtual Reality Might Be the Next Big Thing for Mental Health.* Scientific American Blog Network. https://blogs.scientificamerican.com/observations/virtual-reality-might-be-the-next-big-thing-for-mental-health/.

Medic Alert Advice. (2019, February 24). *Accelerometer: Medical Alert Devices and other interesting applications. Medical Alert Advice.* https://www.medicalalertadvice.com/resources/accelerometer-applications/.

National Institute of Mental Health. (2019, September). *Technology and the Future of Mental Health Treatment.* National Institute of Mental Health. https://www.nimh.nih.gov/health/topics/technology-and-the-future-of-mental-health-treatment/.

O'Hara, D. (2019, June 6). *Wearable technology for mental health*. American Psychological Association. https://www.apa.org/members/content/wearable-technology.

One Mind PsyberGuide. (2021, February 1). *The Mental Health App Guide Designed with You in Mind*. One Mind PsyberGuide. https://onemindpsyberguide.org/.

Palmer, A. (2020, July). *Understanding Stress Using Wearables*. Awake Labs. https://awakelabs.com/reducing-barriers-to-inclusion-wearable-technology/.

Strudwick, G., Impey, D., Torous, J., Krausz, R. M., & Wiljer, D. (2020). Advancing E-Mental Health in Canada: Report From a Multistakeholder Meeting. *JMIR Mental Health, 7*(4). https://doi.org/10.2196/19360

www.ingramcontent.com/pod-product-compliance
Lightning Source LLC
Chambersburg PA
CBHW031429270326
41930CB00007B/636